Principles of Pu

A Simple Text Book on Hy
Principles Fundamental to 1
Individual and Comm

Thomas Dyer Tuttle

Alpha Editions

This edition published in 2024

ISBN 9789362510273

Design and Setting By
Alpha Editions
www.alphaedis.com
Email - info@alphaedis.com

Contents

INTRODUCTION

The earliest history of remote ages describes methods employed in combating disease, and down through all the centuries the struggle against infection has been going on. The science of health as applied in recent years reveals wonderful progress in the avoidance of disease, and in the control of the violent epidemics by which in the past nations were almost exterminated. Modern methods of hygiene and sanitation as applied to public health have robbed smallpox and diphtheria of their death-dealing power; cholera and yellow fever have been forced to retreat before the victorious hosts of applied medical science; tuberculosis, the greatest foe of human life, is slowly but surely receding before the determined efforts of modern preventive medicine.

By nature man is endowed with resistive power sufficient to ward off most forms of disease, provided he keeps his health at a normal standard by right living. If, however, he allows his health to become impaired by reason of overwork, bad habits, wilful exposure to contagion or unhealthful surroundings, he readily falls a prey to disease.

The author of *Principles of Public Health* has here set forth the general rules of life by the observance of which every adult and every child not only can do much to preserve his own health but also can prove himself a prominent factor in raising the standard of public health. A campaign of education is demanded to arrest the enormous loss of life which is carrying so many to untimely graves, and the instruction given in this volume will be of inestimable value in teaching people how to avoid avoidable disease.

The author has not attempted to deal with all the diseases that may be classed as preventable; as the work is intended for use in the public schools, only such diseases are mentioned as it seems fitting to present to school children. To teach our children a proper respect for their own health and for the community welfare is to fit them for the best citizenship.

E. A. PIERCE, M. D.

PORTLAND, OREGON

ACKNOWLEDGMENTS

The author wishes to express his sincere appreciation of the valuable assistance rendered in the preparation of this work by Dr. S. T. Armstrong, of New York City; Dr. H. Wheeler Bond, Commissioner of Health, St. Louis, Missouri; Dr. H. M. Bracken, Secretary and Executive Officer of the State Board of Health of Minnesota; J. S. Caldwell, Professor of Biology, George Peabody College for Teachers, Nashville, Tennessee; R. J. Condon, Superintendent of Schools, Providence, Rhode Island; Mrs. Nona B. Eddy, of the Public Schools of Helena, Montana; Dr. F. M. McMurray, of Teachers College, Columbia University, New York City; Miss Jessie B. Montgomery, Supervising Critic in Training School, State Normal School, Terre Haute, Indiana; Dr. E. A. Pierce, Secretary and Executive Officer of the State Board of Health of Oregon.

PART I
THE FIGHT FOR HEALTH

CHAPTER I

CONSTANT DANGER OF ILLNESS

Every boy and girl confidently expects to grow into a strong and healthy man or woman. How often we hear a child say, "When I am a man," or "When I am a woman;" but I have never heard a boy or a girl say, "If I live to be a man or woman." When you think of what you will do when you are grown into men or women, it never occurs to you that you may be weak and sickly and therefore not able to do the very things that you would most like to do. This suggests that sickness is not natural, else the thought that you may perhaps become sick would enter your mind. As a matter of fact, most sickness is not natural.

The fight for life

There is a constant struggle going on in the world. You see a fight about you every day among the animals. You see the spider catch the fly, the snake catch the frog, the bird catch the insect, and the big fish catch the minnow; and you have heard of wars where men kill one another.

The greatest enemies that men have to fight, however, are not other men, or wild animals, but foes that kill more men, women and children every year than were ever killed in the same length of time by war. These foes are small, very small, but you must not think that because things are small they are not dangerous. We call these foes *disease germs*.

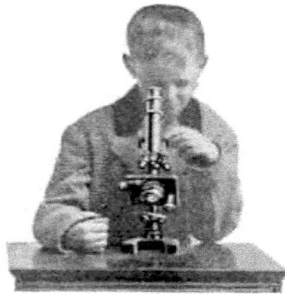

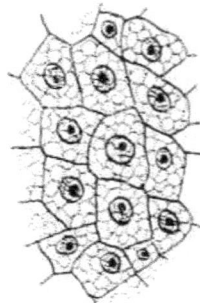

FIG. 1. Looking at cells
through a microscope.

FIG. 2. Some skin cells as seen
through a microscope.

The nature of a germ

The germ is a very, very small body; it is the smallest living body that we know. Later we shall learn that our bodies are made up of cells, and that these cells are extremely small—so small that it takes a very powerful microscope to see one of them. The germ is still smaller than the cells in our bodies, and it is made of a single cell. There are a great many kinds of germs in the world. Fortunately, most of them are not harmful. Some germs cause disease, but there are other germs that not only are not harmful, but are actually helpful to men. Among the helpful germs are those that enrich the ground, and these should be protected; but all germs that cause disease should be destroyed as rapidly as possible. These germs are fighting all the time against our health. They are not armed with guns and cannon, neither do they build forts from which to fight; but they get inside our bodies and attack us there.

How to fight germs

There are three principal ways by which we fight disease germs: *first,* by keeping our bodies so well and strong that germs cannot live in them; *second,* by keeping germs out of our bodies; *third,* by preventing germs from accumulating in the world—that is, by killing as many of them as possible.

If it is possible to keep so well and strong that disease germs cannot live in our bodies, you will naturally infer that there are other causes of sickness besides disease germs. That is true, for there are a great many things beside germs that cause our bodies to get into such a condition that disease germs can enter and grow and make us ill. We sometimes call this a "run-down" condition. Before we begin, then, to study the germs that cause disease, we must learn how to keep our bodies strong and ready to fight these germs.

Questions. 1. What evidence have we that sickness is not natural? 2. Name some of the fights going on in the animal world. 3. What can you say of the amount of illness caused by germs? 4. Tell what you have learned about germs. 5. Name three ways of fighting germs.

Remember. 1. Most sickness comes from failure to observe Nature's laws. 2. We must keep up a constant fight against germs that cause sickness. 3. We fight germs by killing as many of them as we can, and by keeping our bodies so strong that if a disease germ enters it cannot grow.

CHAPTER II

THE NECESSITY OF CARING FOR THE BODY

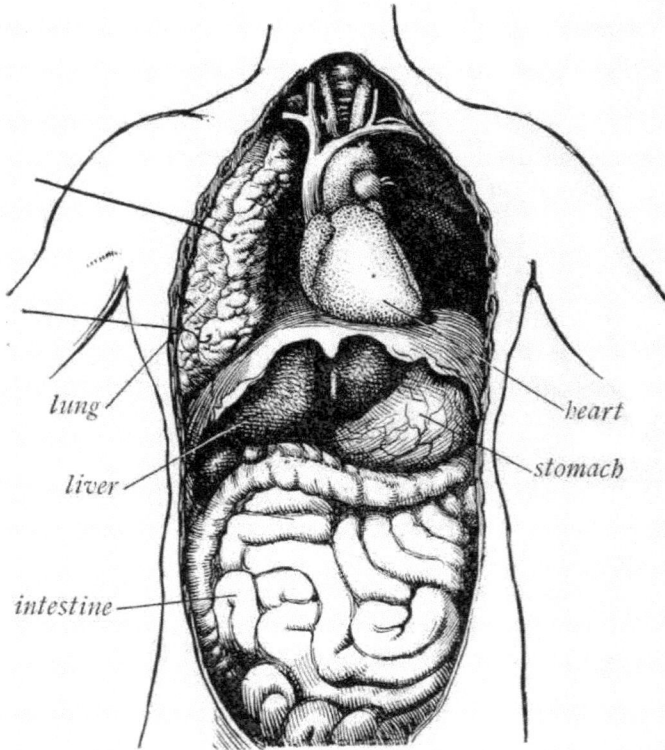

lung

liver

intestine

heart

stomach

FIG. 3. The organs of the body.

How the body is like an automobile

These bodies of ours are built somewhat like automobiles. An automobile is made up of a framework, wheels, body, gasoline tank, engine, and steering-gear. The human body has much the same form of construction. We have a frame, which is made of the bones of the body. We have arms and legs, which correspond to the wheels of the automobile. We have many little pockets in our bodies in which fat is stored, and these little pockets answer to the gasoline tank of the automobile. We have an engine which, like the automobile engine, is made up of many parts; and we have a head or brain, that plays the same part as the steering-gear of the automobile.

The automobile has a tank in which is carried the gasoline necessary to develop power for the machine. If the gasoline gives out, the engine will not run, and before the owner starts on a trip, he is always careful to see that the tank is well filled. In the same way, if we do not provide new fat for the pockets in our bodies in which the fat is stored, our supply will soon give out and our bodies will refuse to work, just as the engine of the automobile will refuse to work when the gasoline is used up.

What cells are like

The automobile is made of iron and wood and rubber, and each bit of iron and wood and rubber is made up of tiny particles. The body is made of bones and muscles, covered with skin, and all these are made up of very fine particles that we call cells. Every part of the body is made of these fine cells. The cells are so small that they can be seen only with a powerful microscope. If you look at your hand you cannot see a cell, because it takes a great many cells to make a spot large enough for you to see. In Figure 1 you see a boy looking through a microscope, and beside him you see a picture of what he sees. This picture does not look like the skin on your hand, neither does it look like the skin on the boy's hand; but it is nothing more nor less than a piece of skin taken from that boy's hand, and it looks just as a piece of skin from your own hand would look if you were to see it through a very strong microscope.

Why cells must not be killed

The whole body is made up of just such little cells as you see in Figure 4, and each cell is alive and has a certain work to perform. It is very important that we keep these cells from dying and that they perform the work for which they are intended, for if these cells die or fail to act, the body becomes sick or dies.

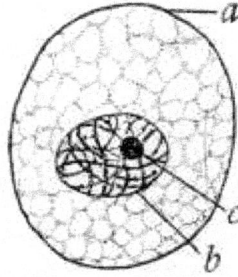

FIG. 4. A cell. (a) Cell body; (b) nucleus; (c) nucleolus.

You can scratch some of the paint from your automobile and the machine will work just as well as ever. Apparently no harm has been done, but an opening has been made through which moisture and germs can enter and cause the wood to rot and the iron to rust. You can remove certain parts of the automobile and still the machine will do its work; but you cannot take away too much of any one part without weakening the automobile, and if certain parts are missing (such as the sparker, the battery, or the steering-gear), the usefulness of the machine is destroyed. So it is with the body. You can scratch off some of the skin and not do any apparent harm, but you have made an opening through which germs may get into the body. You can remove certain parts of the body, such as the arm or leg, and still the body will do efficient service. But there are certain parts of the body that are necessary to life, just as certain parts of the automobile are necessary to the usefulness of the machine. You cannot remove the heart and live; you cannot remove the brain and live.

How cells are killed

You are probably thinking that it must be easy to kill such a little thing as a cell; and so it is. Cells can be killed by too much heat or too much cold. When you skin your hand, you kill many cells, and at the same time make an opening for germs to get in and cause sickness. You can kill cells also by starving them, for they must have not only enough food, but the right kind of food. If you feed your bodies on nothing but candy, pie, and cake, most of the cells will refuse to perform their work and many of them will die. These cells must have also an abundance of air, and the air must be pure and fresh. If you breathe the air that others have breathed or that contains poison of any kind, you will soon find that you are not feeling well. This simply means that so many of the cells are being starved for fresh air, that not enough strong ones are left to do the necessary work. You can kill these cells by overwork, for they must have a proper amount of rest. If you go to school all day long and then sit up until midnight every night, you must not expect the cells of your body to keep strong and well. You can kill these cells by the use of certain things that act as poisons to them, such as tobacco, beer, wine, or whisky.

Questions. 1. In what way is the body like an automobile? 2. What are cells like? 3. Why must cells not be killed? 4. Name five ways by which we kill cells.

Remember. 1. Each part of the body is important to the welfare of the whole body. 2. Each part of the body is made up of very small particles that we call cells; each cell in the body is alive and has a certain work to perform. 3. Cells are very easily weakened and killed. 4. There are five principal ways by which we kill the cells in our bodies: by too much heat or cold; by not giving them the proper kinds of foods; by not giving them enough fresh air; by giving them too much work to do; and by poisoning them.

CHAPTER III

HOW CLOTHING AFFECTS HEALTH

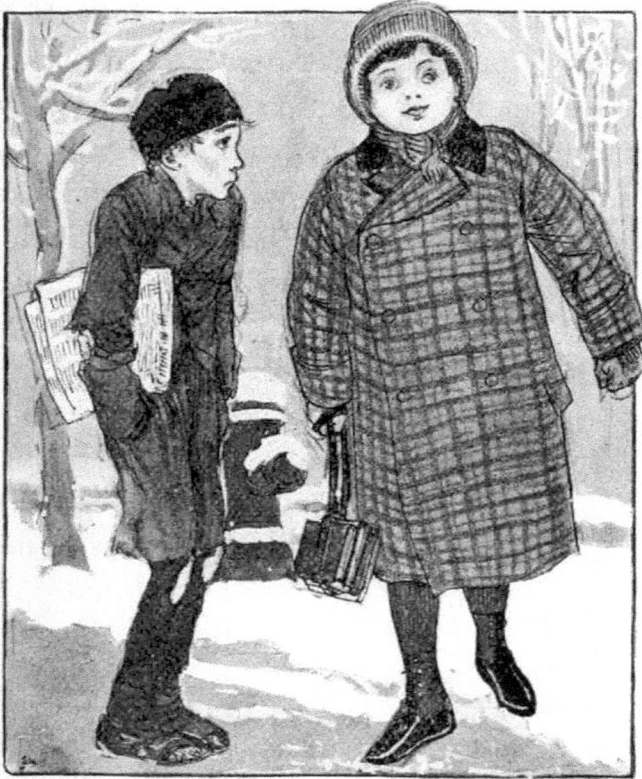

FIG. 5. Warm, dry clothing necessary for health.

Why the body should be equally covered

The body should always be kept at as nearly uniform a temperature as possible. In order to do this we wear clothing. Clothing keeps out the heat on a hot day, just as it keeps the heat in and the cold out on a cold day. The clothing should be equally heavy on all parts of the body. It is not right to wear a thick dress over your chest and leave your shoulders and arms bare, or nearly so. People who do this are killing a great many cells by letting part of their bodies become chilled while the rest is warm, probably too warm.

Why clothing should not be too heavy

The clothing should be just heavy enough to keep the body warm. If you wear such heavy clothing indoors that you are constantly perspiring, your underclothes become damp, and when you go out, even though you put on your overcoat, your body becomes chilled. If you begin to sneeze, that is Nature's way of telling you that you are killing many of your cells by too much cold.

People sometimes get warm from exercising, and then take off their coats. They should have removed their coats before they began to exercise. If you take off your coat after you are too warm, your body becomes chilled. Baseball pitchers know this, and if you watch a good pitcher, you will see that he always puts on his sweater as soon as he stops pitching, even though he is very warm. He knows that if he cools off too quickly, he will become stiff and sore and cannot pitch good ball.

When a draft is dangerous

Sometimes a person sits in a warm room until he begins to perspire freely. Then he opens a window and sits in the draft. Under ordinary conditions, the cool wind alone would chill the body, but now the rapid drying of the perspiration makes the body cool still more quickly. The sudden chill causes the person to take cold, which is simply another way of saying that he has killed many cells and caused others to fall sick, so that they cannot perform their work. We cannot get too much fresh air. Drafts do not hurt us if we are thoroughly wrapped up; but it is very dangerous to allow the wind to strike the body when it is not well protected, and especially when it is damp with perspiration.

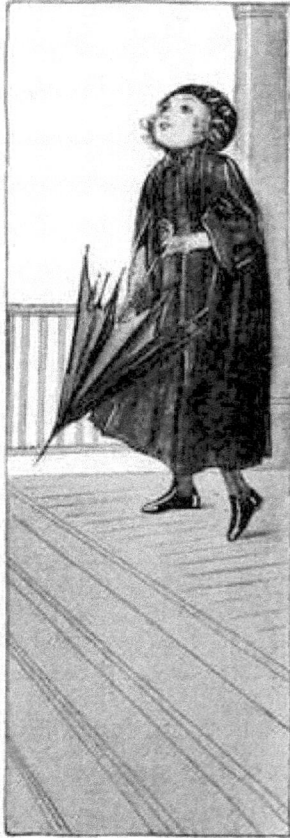

FIG. 6. Properly prepared for wet weather.

Why damp clothing is dangerous

Damp clothing chills the body very rapidly and kills many cells. Indeed, if a single one of the germs that cause pneumonia were to enter your lungs while you were wearing damp clothing, it would grow so rapidly that you might have pneumonia in a very little while. That is why it is important to change your shoes and stockings as soon as you get them wet, and to take off immediately any clothing that becomes damp. It is hard for boys and girls to keep their feet dry in the winter and spring months, and rubbers are a nuisance; but if you expect to grow into the strong man or woman you picture yourself becoming, you must take care to wear your rubbers. Otherwise you may become weak and sickly, and never be able to do the things you hope to do.

The feet are not the only part of the body that needs to be kept dry. A wet coat is just as harmful as wet shoes and stockings; hence, you should always carry an umbrella or wear a raincoat when you go out into the rain. Umbrellas are unhandy for boys and girls to carry, but if you will remember that thousands of little cells in your body are being injured when you get wet and chilled, you will be willing to take your umbrella.

When to wear an overcoat

In cold weather the same amount of clothing should not be worn in the house and outdoors; for this reason, we have overcoats. If you wear your overcoat in the house, you will become overwarm and your underclothing will then become damp with perspiration; when you go outdoors into the cold air, this dampness will have just the same effect as would dampness that comes from outside.

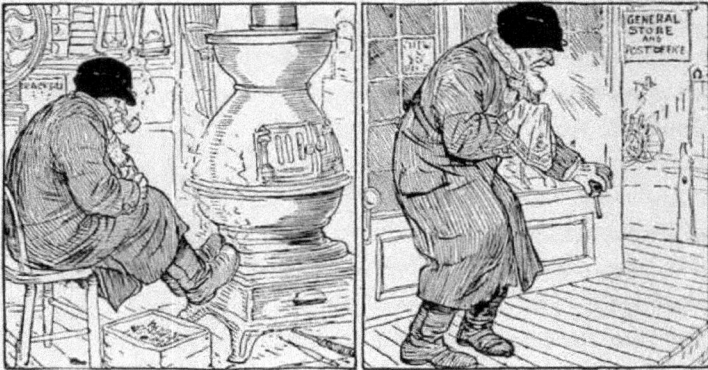

FIGS. 7 and 8. If you keep your overcoat on in the house, your underclothes become damp from perspiration, and when you go outdoors your body becomes chilled.

As soon as the weather gets cold, put on your overcoat every time you go outdoors, and take it off as soon as you come into the house. This is troublesome for boys and girls to do, because they want to run in and out of the house so often; but on the other hand, think of all the cells you will kill if you do not do this, and you will certainly consider it worth while to take off your coat and put it on again.

Questions. 1. How does keeping the body equally covered protect the cells? 2. Give reasons for not wearing too heavy clothing. 3. When is it safe to sit in a draft, and when dangerous? 4. What is the danger of keeping on wet shoes or other damp clothing? 5. When and why should overcoats be worn?

Remember. 1. Clothing should be just heavy enough to keep the body warm all the time. 2. Never take off your coat or sit in a draft when you are too warm. 3. Since wearing damp clothing causes a great deal of sickness, change your clothes as soon as they become wet or damp. 4. Do not forget to take your umbrella when it is raining and to wear your rubbers when the ground is wet. 5. In cold weather wear your overcoat when you are outdoors, but take it off when you come into the house.

CHAPTER IV

THE USES OF FOOD

We kill a great many of the cells in our bodies by starving them; either we do not give them enough food or we do not supply the right kind of food.

Why the body needs new cells

Not only must we feed the cells in our bodies, but we must be constantly making new ones, for in all our work or play, awake or asleep, we are constantly using up certain cells. These cells are used to make the body go, just as the engine uses coal to form the steam that gives it power to run. Boys and girls grow fast and, of course, if they expect to become well men and women, they must make a great many new cells all the time, in addition to those used in doing the work of the body. If we are to make new cells we must have the right kind of food with which to make them.

How the body keeps itself warm

We want to do something besides make new cells; we want to keep warm and well the cells we already have. No amount of clothing would keep you warm if you were not making heat inside your body all the time, any more than you could make a telephone post warm by putting your coat on it. Therefore it is necessary to have food that makes heat in the body, in addition to food that builds cells.

We eat a great many kinds of foods, and all that we eat is used either for building new cells or for producing heat in the body. Thus we can divide all our foods into two classes—building material and heat-producing material. The type of building material is lean meat, and the type of heat-producing material is fat meat and starches, such as potatoes and bread. Milk contains much building material as well as heat-producing material. That is why a baby grows and keeps warm while he takes nothing but milk.

The building foods

Lean meat is the best of all building foods. Eggs are largely a form of lean meat, and hence constitute a good article of food for building purposes. Certain vegetables contain a large per cent of building material; this is especially true of dried beans and peas. Wheat flour and corn meal (particularly when made of whole wheat and unbolted meal) contain much building material.

It is possible for one to live and grow when eating only vegetable matter. But the boy or girl who tries to become a strong man or woman by eating only vegetables will be disappointed; these are mostly heat-producing foods and will not make strong bodies. Experience has proved that the best results are obtained by eating what is called "a mixed diet," that is, a diet composed partly of lean meats and partly of fats and vegetables.

The heat-producing foods

Of the heat-producing foods, fat is the most powerful. Most of the fat that we eat is used immediately for producing in the body heat, and therefore power, but a part of it is stored up for future use. We see it in all healthy young persons. It is this stored-up fat that gives the body its rounded form. When any one has been sick he is thin, because, to produce heat and power while he was sick, he has had to use the fat stored up in his body. To have such a supply of fat is like having a bank account to draw on when out of work. We might call the deposits of fat in our bodies our health banks.

Fat meat is not the only form in which we eat fats; we eat them in a great many other ways. Certain vegetables, such as beans, contain an oil that forms fat. Ripe olives contain a great deal of fatty oil. Butter is a very important form of fat, and cream contains a large amount of it.

Cost of suitable foods

In selecting our foods we should think of two things: *first*, the value of the food as a heat-producer or as a building material; and *second*, the cost of the food. We may like butter much better than bacon, but we should remember that, pound for pound, bacon has a greater nourishing power than butter, and a pound of bacon will cost far less than a pound of butter.

Vegetable foods produce heat by means of the starch which they contain. All vegetables contain starch. This starch is changed into a kind of sugar in the body, and when thus changed it is used to produce heat and power. All vegetable foods do not have the same heat-producing power. There is more heat-producing power in a pound of oatmeal than there is in ten pounds of cabbage. Ten cents' worth of dried beans will produce more heat in the body than will a dollar's worth of lettuce. Thirty cents' worth of corn meal will do more building in the body than will a piece of mutton worth a dollar and a half; but you would have to eat a large amount of corn meal in order to secure the building effect that would result from eating a small quantity of mutton. In most fruits the only nourishing quality is in the sugar they contain. This sugar produces heat in the body just as starch does.

The real value of advertised foods

You will see some foods advertised as possessing a wonderful nourishing power. Do not let such statements deceive you, for no food can have a greater nourishing power than the things from which it is made. If the particular food advertised is made from wheat flour, its nourishing power is just the same as that of an equal quantity of wheat flour. If it is made from corn meal, it can have no greater nourishing power than has the meal itself.

We have learned something about the materials necessary in food and why they are needed. We must now learn why foods that contain these materials sometimes do not give us as good results as we might hope for.

Questions. 1. What use does the body make of new cells? 2. How does the body keep itself warm? 3. Name two uses that the body makes of food. 4. What foods are especially useful for making cells? 5. What foods are chiefly used for making heat? 6. Select articles of food for two meals of equal nourishing value, one meal to be expensive and the other inexpensive. 7. How would you determine the real value of any food?

Remember. 1. Foods are used to make heat and power in the body and to make the body grow. 2. The foods that make the body grow are called building materials, and lean meat is the best kind of building material. 3. The foods that produce heat and power in the body are called heat-producing materials, and fats and starches are the best heat-producers. 4. All vegetables contain starch, some of them contain a fatty oil, and most of them contain some building material. 5. You can get as much building and heat-producing material from cheap foods as you can from expensive foods.

CHAPTER V

CARE OF FOOD—MEATS

Value of meat as a food

Meat is one of the most important articles of our diet. It furnishes essential materials for building cells, and it furnishes fat for making heat and power in the body.

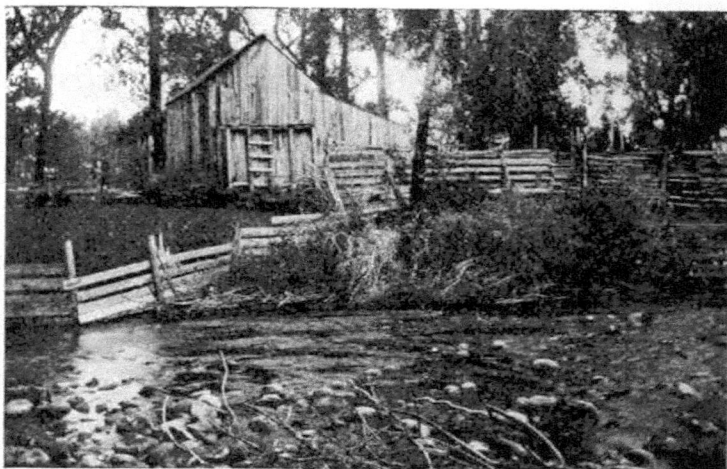

FIG. 9. A double menace to health; the slaughterhouse is dirty, and the filth is drained into a stream.

Characteristics of good meat

Since meat is so important an article of food, we should be very careful to see that it is handled in a way to keep it always perfectly clean. We should make sure that it comes from animals absolutely free from any kind of disease, and that no germs have been allowed to develop poisons in it.

How meat may be kept clean

While people know that they ought to pay attention to these things, as a matter of fact they do not do it. They take very little interest in the way the meat that they are to eat is handled, and very few ever go to the slaughterhouse or into the back room of the butcher shop to see whether things are kept clean or not. Some people say, "Oh, we do not like to go there because it is such a horrid place." If these places were kept clean, as they should be, they would not be "horrid." And if the people who buy the meat would occasionally visit them, these places would be kept clean.

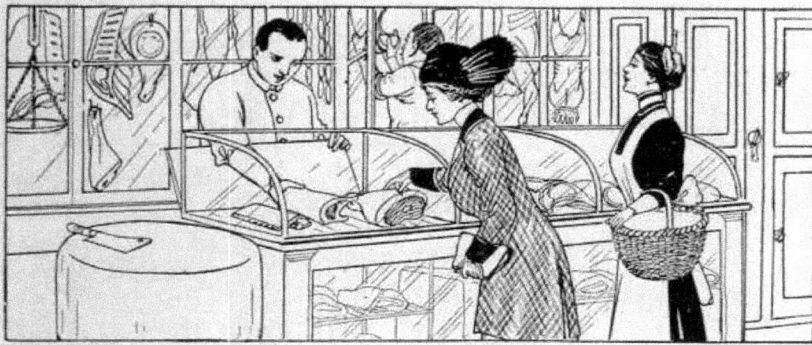

FIG. 10. Properly displayed foods, protected from handling and from dirt and flies.

If the slaughterhouse and the butcher shop where your meats are handled are not kept clean, the meat is sure to have germs growing in it, and these germs will cause poisons called *ptomaines* to form in the meat. There may not be enough of them to make you sick, but there will be enough to injure some of the cells of your body, and to deprive you of much of the nourishment that you would otherwise get from the meat.

All boys and girls should belong to a "Clean Meat League" and should try to persuade their parents not to buy meat from any butcher who does not keep his slaughterhouse and butcher shop clean.

Dangers from diseased meat

Sometimes butchers are anxious to make money fast and take little thought for the number of people they may make ill. They can buy sick cows very much cheaper than well ones. The meat from a sick cow looks just like the meat from a healthy cow, and the dishonest butcher sells both at the same price. The meat from the diseased cow is not suitable for food. It may cause you to have the same disease that the cow had, or it may only be changed to such an extent that it will not give you the nourishment that you should get from good meat. The butcher who sells you meat from a sick cow is of course dishonest.

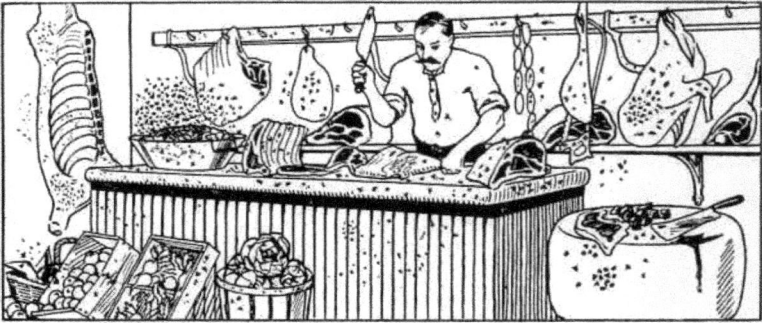

FIG. 11. Improperly displayed foods, exposed to handling and to dirt and flies.

How to prevent the sale of diseased meats

Ask your father to visit the slaughterhouse where your meat is killed. The only thing you need to do is to persuade him to go and see whether the cattle are sick or not. If the cattle look sick, you will not have to ask him not to buy the meat. No person should ever eat meat that comes from a diseased animal, no matter what the nature of the sickness may be. People who will take the trouble to visit the slaughterhouses occasionally, to investigate these things for themselves, will not have such meat offered them.

Importance of giving animals clean food

Animals that are fed on filthy food are not fit for human consumption. Butchers often feed the offal (the insides) of animals to the hogs. This makes the hogs fatten quickly, but it also makes them diseased. When you go to the slaughterhouse with your father, ask him to go around to the back door, and if you see hogs eating this filth, do not buy any more meat from that butcher.

Questions. 1. What use does the body make of meat? 2. What conditions are essential for good meat? 3. How can meat be kept clean? 4. Why is meat from a diseased animal unfit for food? 5. How can you help in preventing the sale of meat from diseased animals? 6. Why should animals not be fed with offal?

Remember. 1. Meat that is not handled in a clean manner is sure to contain germs that cause a poison to form in the meat. 2. Never buy meat from a butcher who does not keep his slaughterhouse and butcher shop clean. 3. Meat from a diseased animal is not fit for food.

4. Meat from animals fed on filthy food should not be eaten. 5. Form a "Clean Meat League" and visit the slaughterhouse where your meat is killed.

CHAPTER VI

CARE OF FOOD—MILK

Milk is another important article of food. The Department of Agriculture at Washington says that milk furnishes sixteen per cent of the nourishment of the people of the country. Milk is an excellent food when it is pure, but when it is not pure it is very dangerous.

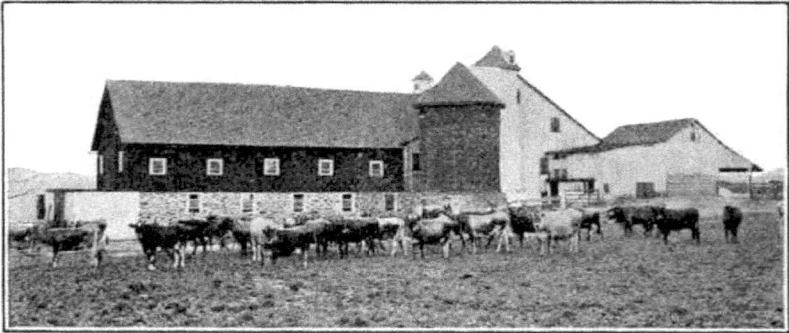

FIG. 12. A clean dairy.

Milk as a carrier of germs

Milk has carried the germs of every disease of which the germ is known; it has also carried many diseases of which we do not know the germ. Disease germs grow rapidly in milk, and they do not make the milk look different or taste different from milk that is perfectly pure. If you could take two bottles of milk entirely free from disease germs and put typhoid fever germs in one, and should set both bottles in an ice box for twenty-four hours, you would not then be able to tell into which one you had put the germs. The milk in both bottles would look and taste just the same. The only difference between the milk in the two bottles would be that if you drank from one it would make you stronger and would furnish you with both building material and power-producing material, while if you drank from the other you would become very ill and would probably die.

How disease germs get into milk:

Since we cannot tell from the taste or the appearance of milk whether or not there are disease germs in it, we must take every precaution possible to keep them out. The first step is to learn where the disease germs come from and how they get into the milk.

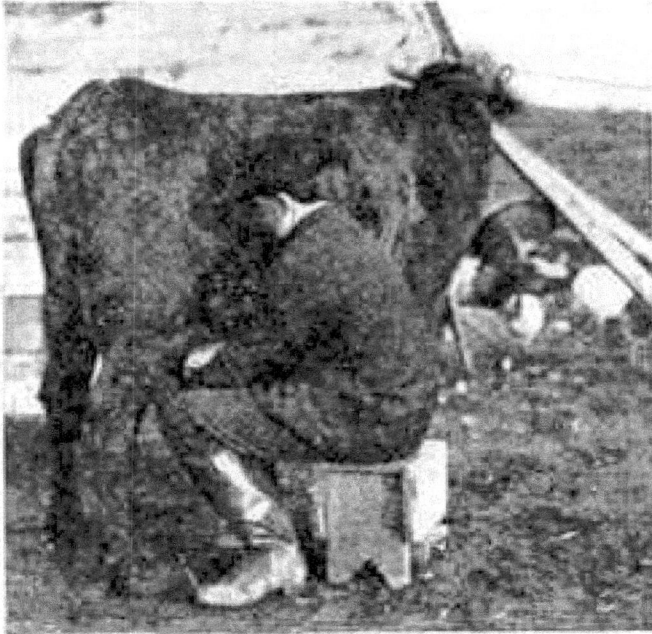

FIG. 13. Polluted milk is sure to come from a dairy where cleanliness is not observed.

(1) By dirt on the cow

Every cow has more or less dirt on her sides and udder; some have a great deal. When the cow is milked, much of the dirt falls into the milk bucket. This dirt always contains a great many germs of different kinds, and many of them are germs that cause disease. Straining the milk will take out much of the dirt, but disease germs will go through the finest strainer that was ever made.

In Figure 13 we see a man milking a dirty cow. The owner has allowed his lot to become so dirty that the cow cannot find a clean place in which to lie down. If the man kept his lot clean, and if before milking the light dirt on the cow's sides and udder were wiped off with a damp cloth, no germs would fall into the milk.

Another source of dirt and disease germs in milk is the barn. The walls of a barn where cows are milked should always be kept clean and should be whitewashed frequently. If this is done, there will be comparatively little dirt on the walls to fall into the milk.

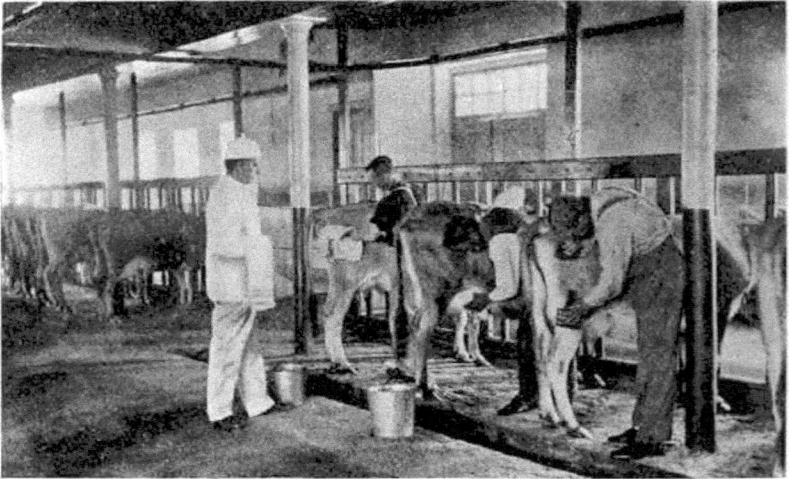

FIG. 14. Only clean milk will come from a dairy where proper precautions are taken.

Of course the walls and floors of a barn cannot be kept absolutely clean. There will always be some dirt, and the movements of the cows shifting their position and switching their tails, will stir up the dust; so it is important to remove the milk from the barn as soon as possible. Milk cans should never be kept in the barn. The milk should be taken directly from the barn to a cooling house and there strained.

All barns where cows are kept should have plenty of windows, that there may be an abundance of light and fresh air. Cows need fresh air just as much as people do, while a barn that is not supplied with plenty of light is very likely to be a dirty barn.

Keep dirt and disease germs out of the milk by keeping the barn clean and by taking the milk away from the barn as soon as possible.

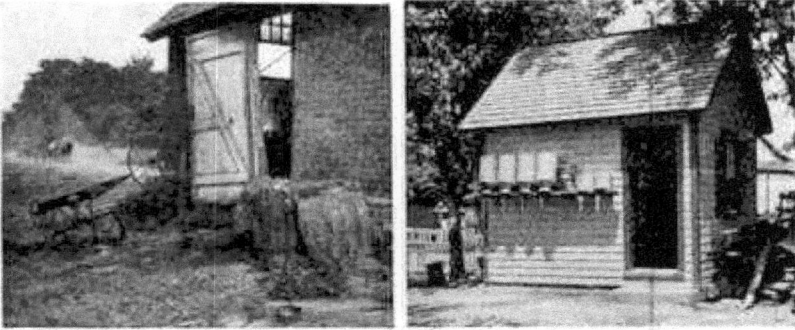

FIG. 15. A dirty, insanitary milk-house.

FIG. 16. A clean, inexpensive milk-house.

(3) By dirt on the milkman

Another source of dirt and disease germs in milk is the milkman or milkmaid. No matter how careful we may be, our clothes hold more or less dust, and all dust contains germs, very often disease germs. When a person is milking a cow, the dust from his clothes is shaken off into the milk. The only way to avoid this is to wear, while milking, a special suit of clothes made of white cloth, which may be washed as soon as it shows the least particle of dirt.

The milker's hands, too, are often dirty. Perhaps he carefully washes his hands after milking, but not before. It is a common custom for milkers to moisten their hands with milk while milking, and to do this frequently. The result is that dirty milk from their hands is constantly dropping into the milk pail. This is a very bad habit, and doubly bad if the milkman has not washed his hands before milking.

Sometimes there are sick people at the dairy farm. Often some one nurses a sick person until milking time and then goes out and milks the cows. When this is done, the milker is almost sure to plant the germs of the disease in the milk. No milk should ever be used from any dairy where there is an infectious disease; and no one who has charge of a sick person, no matter what the nature of the sickness, should ever handle milk that is to be used by others.

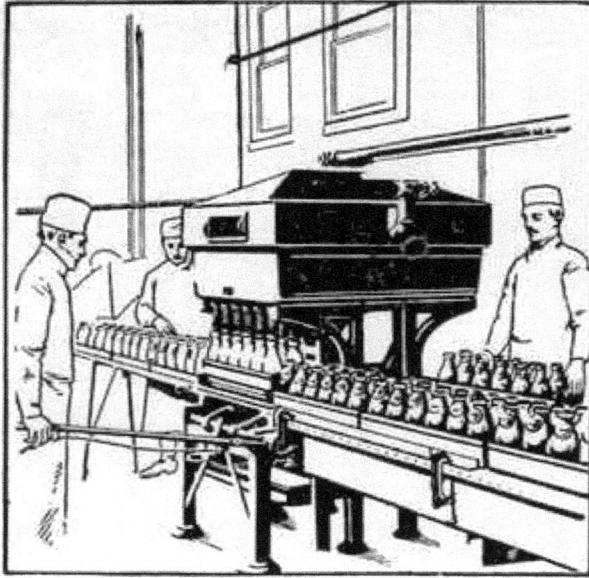

FIG. 17. A model bottling establishment.

(4) By dirt in cans and bottles

The cans and bottles in which the milk is placed are frequently sources of dirt and germs. Milk cans and bottles are supposed to be thoroughly washed before milk is put into them, and they should be thoroughly scalded after they are washed. This is not always done, and sometimes the bottles are not washed at all.

Some dairymen will tell you that the bottles and cans are always washed and scalded just before the milk is put into them, and that this is never neglected by any dairyman. That is what a dairyman once told me. Then I asked him how he accounted for the fact that I had found a milk ticket in the bottle with the fresh milk. Of course he could not explain this, though I thought I could explain it for him. The old milk bottle was returned to the milkman with the ticket for the new milk inside it. The deliveryman left the fresh milk, but forgot to take the ticket out of the bottle; and the man who "washed" the bottles must have forgotten to take out the ticket too. Of course, the bottle was not washed at all, and if one bottle goes unwashed, it is reasonable to assume that others are neglected in the same way.

Milk bottles and cans should always be thoroughly washed before fresh milk is put into them. This washing cannot be done by little children; it is work for a man or woman, and careful work at that.

(5) By polluted water

I have just told you that milk vessels should be thoroughly washed. It is true, however, that disease germs may get into the milk through this very process of washing the vessels. Water sometimes contains disease germs, especially the germs that cause typhoid fever, cholera, and other diseases of the intestines. Such water is said to be polluted. When milk vessels are washed with polluted water, the germs are left in them and thus get into the milk. If the water used to wash the cans is thoroughly boiled, the germs will be killed; hence it is important to scald all milk vessels.

All water used about a dairy should be perfectly pure. If there is the least suspicion about the quality of the water, it should be examined by a chemist; and if it is not pure, the milk from such a dairy should not be used. In order to prevent the possibility of any infection, all water used to wash milk vessels should be thoroughly boiled even when the water is known to be pure, and the vessels should afterward be scalded, to kill any germs that may be left after washing.

(6) By flies falling into the milk

Flies very frequently get into the milk. Later we shall learn more about how flies carry germs, but at present it is enough to know that on every fly there are a great many germs, and whenever a fly gets into milk it plants those germs and they grow very rapidly. As soon as a cow is milked, the milk should be taken to a clean cooling house, with screens at all the windows and doors, and there strained into a vessel and cooled.

(7) By disease in the cow

The last way that we will mention by which germs get into milk is by disease in the cow herself. Cows suffer from many diseases, just as men do; and when a cow is sick, her milk is very likely to contain the germs of the disease that is making her sick. Especially is this true of tuberculosis, or consumption, as it is called. A great many children get consumption by drinking milk from consumptive cows. No milk should ever be used from a cow that is not healthy. All dairy cows should be examined at frequent intervals by a competent veterinarian to make sure that they are free from any disease.

Questions. 1. Milk forms what per cent of the food of the people of the United States? 2. Why is it important that milk should be kept clean? 3. Name some ways by which germs get into milk. 4. What is the danger from a dirty cow and barn? 5. How can this danger be prevented? 6. How does the milkman allow germs to get into the milk, and how can he avoid doing so? 7. How should milk cans and bottles be washed? 8. Why is it important that only pure water be used about the dairy? 9. How can flies be kept out of milk? 10. How should milch cows be tested to make sure that they are free from tuberculosis?

Remember. 1. Milk is a very important article of food; it is both a building and a heat-producing material. 2. When milk is not properly handled, it contains many disease germs. 3. Disease germs often get into milk from unwashed bottles and cans; from dirty barns; from dirty milkmen; from dirty water used to wash the cans and bottles; from flies falling into the milk; from diseased cows.

CHAPTER VII

DECOMPOSITION OF FOOD

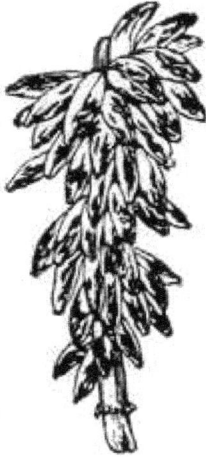

FIG. 18. Partially decayed fruit is not fit for food.

Why partially decomposed foods should not be eaten

Vegetables and fruits that are partially decayed should not be eaten. Even if an orange is decayed only on one side, the products of decomposition—that is, the poisons produced by decay—have extended all through the orange. You cannot see them, but they are there. It is the same with a decaying apple, potato, or melon. It never pays to buy partially decayed or stale fruits or vegetables, for not only are they dangerous to health, but they are so reduced in nourishing qualities by decomposition that you get little value for the money you spend. It is always better economy to buy fresh fruits and vegetables, or even canned vegetables, when the latter are properly put up.

What causes decomposition

All decomposition (rotting) in fruits and vegetables is due to the action of germs. If you will look at a bunch of old grapes, you will notice that some of the grapes are rotten, while others have dried up. Now, if you examine them very carefully, you will find that all the decomposed grapes have breaks in the skin. The break may be very small, but it is there, and through this break the germs that cause decomposition have entered. You will find also that there is not the slightest break in the skin of any grape that has dried up. The germs could not enter, hence there has been no decomposition. It is the same with other fruits and vegetables: if the germs that cause decomposition cannot get inside, the fruit or vegetable will dry up, but will not rot.

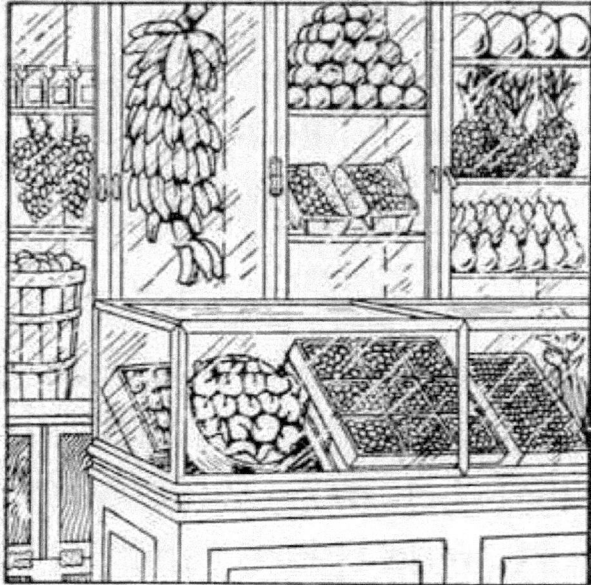

FIG. 19. Fruits displayed for sale, but properly protected from flies, dust, and dirty hands.

Germs can go through a very small opening—so small that you may not be able to find it; but if there is decomposition, the hole is there.

The skin of the body acts in the same way as the skin of the grape and keeps out a great many germs that would make us sick were they able to get through the skin. They often get through the skin when we cut ourselves.

Meats decompose as well as fruits and vegetables, and the decomposition is due to the presence of germs in the meat. We cannot keep all germs out of meat, but we can keep out a great many of them by having everything clean about the meat, by keeping it covered as much of the time as possible, and by handling it only with clean hands.

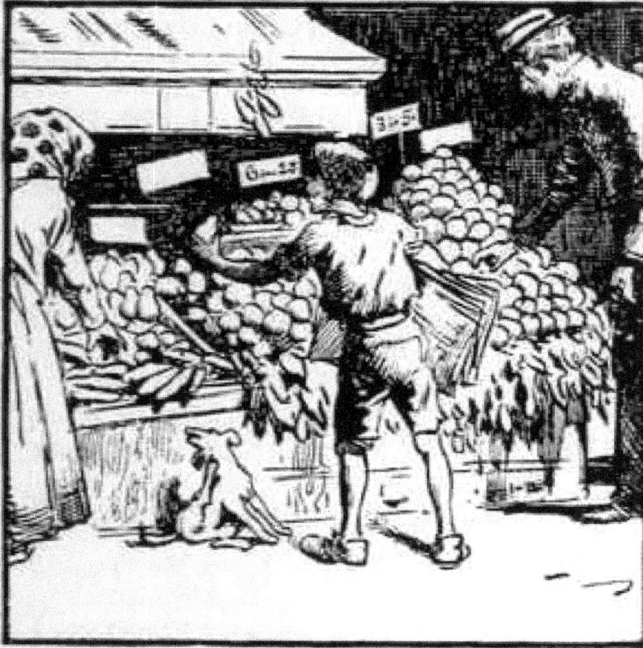

FIG. 20. Fruits for sale, not properly protected from flies, dirt, and other sources of filth.

Why foods do not decompose in very cold places

When meat is kept so cold that it is almost frozen, the germs cannot grow, and decomposition is prevented. In this way meat can be kept perfectly free from decomposition for several weeks. After the meat is taken from the cold storage room, it should be cut as soon as possible into steaks, roasts, and other pieces for cooking; and when taken to your home, it should be kept in an ice box until the time to cook it. You cannot keep meat very long at home without decomposition starting, because small ice boxes are not cold enough to check entirely the growth of germs.

Unless the meat is to be eaten hot, it should be cooled after cooking and placed again in the ice box as soon as possible. Cooking kills the germs that are in the meat before it is cooked; but unless it is kept in a very cold place and protected from flies after it is cooked, germs will get into it again as soon as it is cold. Cooked meat will decompose just the same as uncooked meat.

What is formed in food by decomposition

When germs are allowed to grow in meat, as always happens when it is not kept in a very cold place, these germs cause the poisons that we call ptomaines. The people who eat such meat become sick, and in many cases do not recover. Cooking meat that contains ptomaines will kill the germs that caused the poison, but it will not destroy the poison that has already been formed.

Why some canned meats are poisonous

People not infrequently are poisoned by eating canned meat. Sometimes you will hear it said that the poison formed because the meat was in cans. This is not true; the cans had nothing to do with the forming of the poison. This was caused by germs that were allowed to grow in the meat before it was cooked. When the meat was cooked the germs were killed, but the poison was not destroyed. In other words, the poison developed before the meat was canned, and not after it was put into the cans.

Questions. 1. What is the objection to eating fruits when they are partially decayed? 2. Why do some foods shrivel while others decay? 3. Why does decomposition not go on in cold places? 4. What are ptomaines? 5. When are ptomaines formed in canned meats?

Remember. 1. Partially decomposed fruits or vegetables are not suitable for foods. 2. Meats in which germs have been allowed to grow should not be eaten. 3. Cooking meat kills the germs in it, but does not destroy the poisons that the germs have formed. 4. When canned meats are poisonous, it is because the poison was formed before the meat was canned; the poison is not caused by the can.

CHAPTER VIII

HARM DONE BY IMPROPER COOKING

Nearly all food should be cooked before it is eaten; but if the cooking is not properly done, much of the nourishing power of the food is destroyed, and in some instances the food is rendered actually injurious.

Why starchy foods should be thoroughly cooked

Starchy foods should be thoroughly cooked in order that the coverings which surround the little granules may be broken or made soft. If starchy foods are not thoroughly cooked, the little grains go into the stomach as hard as grains of sand; then most of them are not digested at all, but pass out of the system without furnishing any nourishment to the body. If starchy foods are fried in fats, as is the case with doughnuts, the granules of starch become coated with fat. As the fat is not digested until it comes to the intestines, the saliva never reaches the coverings of the starch, and more work is thrown on the other juices of the body. The result is that the little glands which make these other juices are overworked, or else the starch is not digested at all and therefore furnishes no nourishment to the body. When bread is sticky (we sometimes call it soggy) in the middle of the loaf, it is because the flour has not been thoroughly cooked and the little grains or granules of starch are still hard. You cannot feel these granules between your fingers, but they are hard just the same, and very little of such food is made use of in the body.

Remember that all starchy foods should be thoroughly cooked, and remember, too, that all vegetables are chiefly starchy in character.

How fats should be cooked

When fats are cooked over a very hot fire, an acid is developed that is injurious to the body. This does not mean that when the fire is hot enough to broil a steak well, it causes this acid to form; neither does it mean that heat sufficient to boil the grease for cooking doughnuts will cause it to form. Every cook knows that when she fries fat meat over a fire that is too hot, it has a bitter taste. This bitter taste is caused by an acid which will destroy a part of the usefulness of the food in the body and will cause many of the cells to stop doing their work properly.

How meats should be cooked

There is a great difference of opinion in regard to cooking foods, especially meats. Some people will tell you that meats should not be cooked at all; that man originally ate his meat raw and that this is the proper way. Others will tell you that all meat should be cooked until it does not show a particle of red, even until it is dry throughout. These are the two extremes; and it is never well to go to extremes in anything, especially in matters that concern the health.

Meat should always be cooked, because by being cooked it is made more easily digestible; but it should not be cooked, until all the juices, which contain much of the nourishing matter, are dried up and the meat made hard. Meat that is cooked until it is dry and hard is more difficult to digest than meat that is not cooked at all.

Questions. 1. What effect has improper cooking on foods? 2. Why should starches be thoroughly cooked? 3. What is the objection to starchy foods fried in grease? 4. What changes take place in fatty food when it is fried over a very hot fire? 5. Why should all meats be cooked? 6. What is the objection to cooking meat until the juices are dried out?

Remember. 1. Starchy foods should be thoroughly cooked so that the fine grains may be softened and the food thus made more easy to digest. 2. Fats should not be fried over a very hot fire because too much heat causes a poison to form in the fat. 3. Meats should be cooked, but never until they become dry, as the juices in the meat contain most of the nourishing material.

CHAPTER IX

HOW NEATNESS, CHEERFULNESS, AND GOOD MANNERS PROMOTE HEALTH

Why mealtime should be pleasant

The dining table should be the pleasantest and most inviting place in the house. If you are complaining and quarreling during the meal, you cannot enjoy the food; you cannot eat it properly; and your ill temper will so affect your body that you cannot properly digest what you eat. A dirty table, with flies swarming over the food, is not very tempting, and when seated at such a table, one does not eat the things that are best for him and sometimes does not eat anything at all.

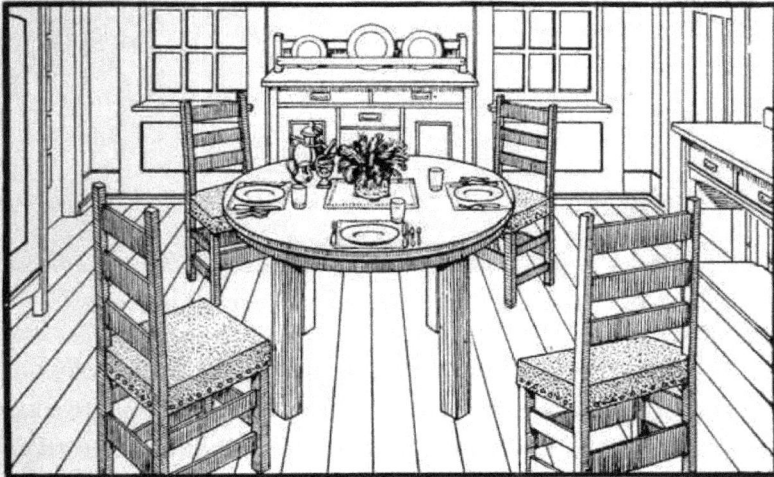

FIG. 21. A clean, inviting dining-room.

How uninviting luncheons affect the appetite

The luncheons that boys and girls take to school with them are often prepared in so careless a way that they are extremely uninviting. The substantial school lunch can be made just as appetizing as the dainty refreshments at an afternoon tea or at a party. If the same care is devoted to the preparation of the one as of the other, boys and girls will eat their lunches with enjoyment and good appetites.

Why an attractive table calls for pleasing guests

If the table is made to look clean and inviting, do you not think that you, in your turn, should make yourself as neat and clean as possible before you come to it? Dirt on your hands and face not only does not look well, but contains a great many germs that may get into your food and thus find their way into your body and try to make you ill.

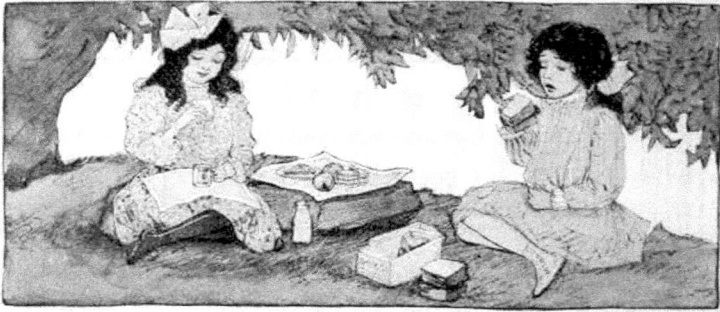

FIG. 22. Two lunches. Which is the more tempting?

How foods should be eaten

Besides being eaten in pleasant surroundings, all food should be eaten slowly. Let us suppose that we are all seated at a clean, inviting table and everyone is clean and happy. Before the children is the very kind of food that is best for them. It looks good and they know it is good, and they want to eat all they can of it. But they think of a game of jacks or of ball that they want to play as soon as dinner is over, so they simply "bolt" their food.

What are teeth made for? Why, to chew with, of course. But why are we given some teeth that are sharp like knives, and some that are flat like millstones? It seems probable that these different kinds of teeth are intended for special purposes, and so they are. If our teeth were intended only for cutting our food into bits small enough to swallow without causing pain, there would be no need for any except the sharp, knife-like teeth. But we have the big grinders, which were made to use, and it is very important that they be used in the right way.

Why food should be thoroughly chewed

We do not chew our food simply to make it fine enough to swallow, but for quite another reason as well. In our mouths there is a fluid called *saliva*. Think of something that you are very fond of eating, and the mere thought of it makes the saliva come into your mouth. This saliva has a very important duty to perform in connection with preparing the food for the little cells of the body. Each little grain of starch—and you will remember that all vegetable foods are composed largely of starch—has a capsule about it. This simply means that it is done up in a little package. The saliva helps to open this capsule by making it soft (just as water will soften the paper on a package of candy), so that the other digestive juices can reach the starch and turn it into the kind of sugar that is used in the body. If you do not chew your food very fine, the saliva will not reach the starch granules, the little packages of starch will be hard to open when they go into the stomach, and much of the starch will never be made use of in the body. The saliva has much the same action on the coverings of the little packages of meat, for all the meat that we eat is done up in similar packages.

A great Englishman, Mr. Gladstone, who lived to be eighty-three, made a practice of chewing every bite of food twenty times, and he thought this had a great deal to do with his being such a strong and well man and living to such an old age.

When desserts are not harmful

After you have eaten meats, bread, and vegetables, it will do no harm to eat a piece of pie or cake, or a dish of ice-cream or some other dessert. It is not easy, as a rule, to digest these things (that is, to get them into such shape that they can be used as food by the little cells in the body), but a moderate amount of them is very good for boys and girls, as well as for grown people. If you refuse to eat the meat and bread, but wait until the dessert is served and then fill your stomach with sweet things, you will be starving some of the little cells, and you will be reminded of this very soon. Sometimes you may be reminded of it by having a pain in your stomach, but more often by getting low grades in your lessons at school. Your teacher will know it, too, because you will be so restless and inattentive in your classes that she will have to give you a low grade in deportment as well.

Questions. 1. What kind of topics should be discussed at mealtime? 2. What is the objection to an untidy table? 3. What kind of luncheon do you like best? 4. What does a clean table call for? 5. What is the importance of eating slowly? 6. Why should we chew our food thoroughly? 7. When are desserts not harmful?

Remember. 1. The dining table should be the most inviting place in the house. 2. Unpleasant subjects should be avoided at mealtime. 3. A clean table calls for clean people. 4. Eat slowly and chew your food thoroughly, that the saliva may reach each grain of starch. 5. Desserts are not harmful if eaten at the end of a meal composed of good building and heat-producing materials.

CHAPTER X

DANGERS FROM POOR TEETH

We have learned that chewing is not merely a process of cutting our food into such lumps as we can swallow without hurting ourselves; but that the food must be ground up fine and thoroughly mixed with the saliva, that the saliva may reach every particle of starch. If we do not have good teeth, we cannot grind our food as fine as it ought to be ground, and, as a result, a great deal of the starch will not be reached by the saliva.

Nature starts every child with a full set of good, strong, clean teeth. These teeth, which we call first, or milk, teeth, are not very large, but they are perfect in every respect and last until the second, or permanent, teeth come in. That is, they will last so long *if they are taken care of.* If they are not taken care of, they will decay just as the later teeth will decay, and they must be cared for in the same way.

Why we have baby or milk teeth

Boys and girls sometimes wonder why they have a set of teeth that come out before they can have the teeth that must last them the rest of their lives. This is simply because there is not room enough in a child's mouth for the big, permanent teeth. We must have teeth while our jaws are growing, so we have first a set of little teeth. Then just as soon as our jaws get large enough for the big teeth, the little teeth come out and the big ones come in.

Teeth are about the hardest substance in the body. If we take care of our second teeth, they should last as long as we live. The only reason they do not last is because we do not take care of them. If a person would keep his teeth clean all the time, he would rarely be obliged to have a single permanent tooth pulled.

Why teeth break easily

Teeth are so hard that they are brittle, that is, they break easily. Glass is brittle, and you can chip off a piece of glass with a pin by sticking the pin into a crack in the glass. In just the same way you can chip off a piece of a tooth by sticking a pin between two teeth. That is what often happens when people pick their teeth with pins, or with any other hard substance. A metal toothpick is just as bad as a pin.

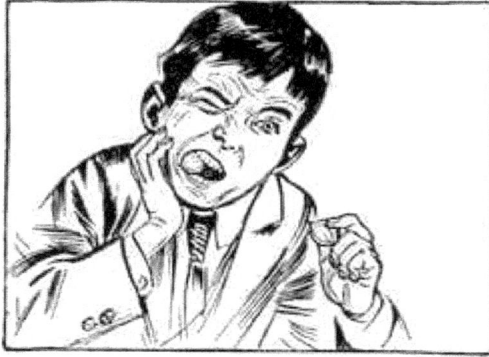

FIG. 23. Teeth were not intended for nutcrackers.

Another way by which little pieces are chipped off the teeth is by biting hard things. Sometimes we see boys and girls cracking nuts with their teeth; again we see them trying to bite wires in two. They put their teeth to many uses for which teeth were never made. They do not realize, while they are abusing their teeth in this way, that they are probably chipping the enamel, which is the hard, shiny covering of the tooth, and are destroying the one protection that their teeth have against decay.

Why teeth decay

When a little piece is chipped off a tooth, an opening is made through the enamel. Through this opening germs may lodge in the inner part of the tooth, which is soft. When this happens, a little black speck appears on the tooth, and after a while the tooth begins to ache. If you have a toothache, you go to a dentist, and he probably finds that germs have caused the tooth to decay until there is a hole extending into the very center of it.

Teeth grow very close together, but there is always a little space between them. Whenever you eat anything, particles of the food get into these spaces and if allowed to remain there, soon decompose. These decomposing particles of food between the teeth will gradually soften even the enamel, and in this way little openings are made for germs to get into the teeth.

How to care for the teeth

Never pick the teeth. You cannot make them clean by picking them. Every morning and night brush your teeth with a stiff toothbrush and a little tooth powder. Brush them both crosswise and up and down, to get out everything from between them. Do not think you have done your duty if you brush only your front teeth, the ones that show. Brush the back teeth just as thoroughly as you do the front teeth. Very few people will see your back teeth, but these decay just as fast as your front teeth, if they are not kept clean.

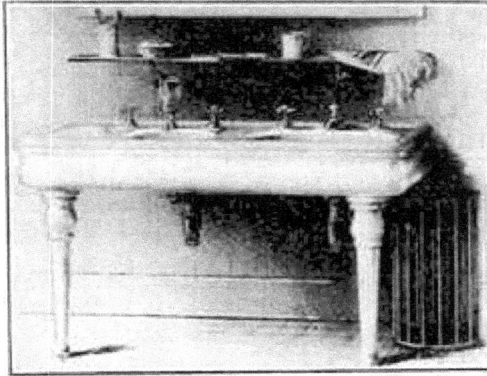

FIG. 24. A sanitary wash-basin with a separate bowl for washing the teeth.

How often one should go to the dentist

Twice each year you should have a dentist examine your teeth, to see if there are any little spots where decay has started. If you have kept your teeth perfectly clean all the time, and have not chipped off little pieces, there will be none of these decayed spots. But it is a safe plan to have the teeth looked over at least twice a year, for you may have broken a tooth without knowing it, and by the time a decayed spot is large enough to cause pain, or has made a hole that you can feel with your tongue, it has advanced much farther than it should have been permitted to do.

Questions. 1. Why should you chew your food thoroughly? 2. Why is it necessary to have baby teeth? 3. How are teeth easily broken? 4. Why do teeth decay? 5. What must you avoid in order to protect your teeth? 6. How should your teeth be brushed? 7. Why should you have your teeth examined twice each year by a dentist?

Remember. 1. Take care of your teeth and they will last you as long as you live. 2. Do not pick them with pins, or toothpicks of any kind. 3. Do not use them for nutcrackers or wire-cutters. 4. Do not use them for tack pullers. 5. Keep them clean at all times. 6. Brush them up and down as well as crosswise.

CHAPTER XI

NECESSITY FOR PURE AIR AND HOW TO SECURE IT

We have learned how the cells of the body are killed by starvation. Now let us learn how they are choked to death, or killed by lack of air.

How air is changed in the body

The cells of the body need *oxygen*, and the only way we can give it to them is by means of air. Every time we take air into our lungs we are giving oxygen to the red corpuscles or cells in the blood, which distribute it to the other cells in the body. The air that goes into our lungs, if it is fresh and pure, contains a great deal of oxygen and a very little of another gas called *carbon dioxid*. The air that comes out of the lungs contains a very little oxygen and a great deal of carbon dioxid. The blood not only takes the oxygen out of the air, but gives carbon dioxid to the air. This carbon dioxid is very poisonous, and would kill the cells if it remained in the blood; hence we should never breathe the same air twice. There is no lack of fresh air in the world, and no excuse for anyone's ever breathing air that is not pure.

Effects of impure air

If you close all the windows and doors in the schoolroom and shut up the ventilators, you will soon find that you are not able to pay close attention to your studies, and in a little while you will begin to feel drowsy. This is because you have used up so much of the oxygen in the air that there is no longer enough to supply the demands of the little cells, and because, in addition, you are taking into your bodies the poisonous carbon dioxid that has been breathed out into the room. It takes a great deal of fresh air to supply the body with oxygen—about 1,250 cubic feet of air each hour. With thirty or forty children in a room, it does not take long to use up all the oxygen. So there should be a constant supply of fresh air coming into the room.

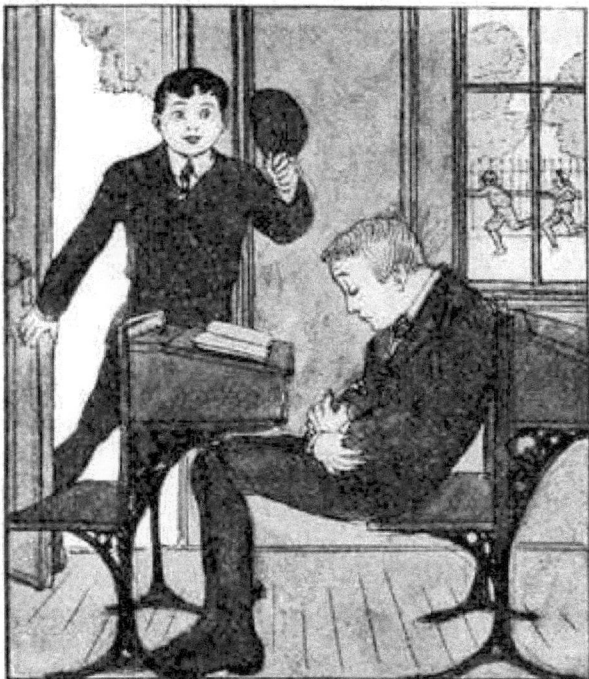
FIG. 25. Results of breathing good and bad air.

Methods of ventilation

It is not only in the schoolroom that you need oxygen. When you are out-of-doors you get an abundance of fresh air, but from a great many houses every bit of fresh air is shut out. It is always possible to let an abundance of fresh air into any house without causing a draft. A piece of board can be made to fit into a window frame so that when the window is raised, the air will be directed upward and will not cause a draft. Hot-air furnaces are made with cold-air pipes. The fresh air from outdoors comes through these cold-air pipes and, after being heated, is driven into the rooms of the house. Some people think they will save coal by closing these drafts. Not only do they not save coal (for the furnace does not give as much heat when this draft is closed), but they kill their body cells by refusing to give them oxygen. The cold-air pipe in a hot-air furnace should always be kept wide open.

In houses heated with steam or hot water, either the windows must be kept open, or some other way must be provided for admitting fresh air and taking out foul air. These arrangements constitute a system of ventilation.

Houses heated with stoves must also be provided with some means of ventilation. The stove, by its draft, takes out a little of the foul air, but it will not take out more air than one person poisons.

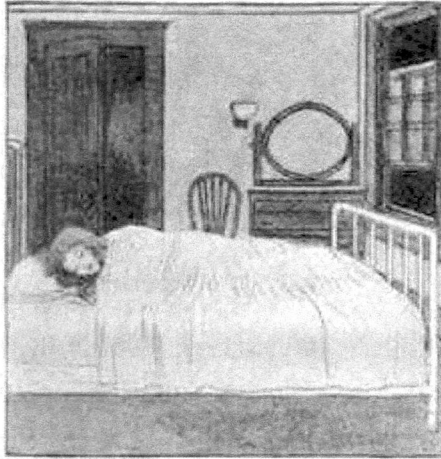

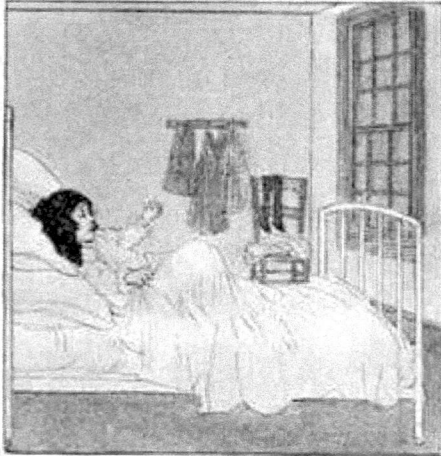

FIG. 26. Restfulness: Effect of good ventilation in a sleeping-room, with the right position for sleeping.

FIG. 27. Restlessness: Effect of poor ventilation in a sleeping-room, with the wrong position for sleeping.

Why windows should be kept open at night

Many people seem to think that they do not need fresh air at night, and they close their bedroom windows as tight as they can. Those people do not sleep well and often have bad colds. You should always sleep with your windows open. If it is impossible for you to have your windows open without having a draft, choose the draft; it will do you no harm if you are well covered, and under no circumstances will it do you as much harm as the foul air that you breathe if your window is closed. Some persons (fortunately they are few nowadays) will tell you that night air is dangerous. I wonder what kind of air these people expect to breathe at night. Do they expect to fill the room in the daytime with enough air for use at night? Such air would certainly not be very fresh. Night air is the only kind of air that it is possible to breathe at night.

The ventilation of public assembly rooms

Churches, theaters, and ten-cent shows are often very poorly ventilated. You can always tell a poorly ventilated room by the foul odor when you go into it from the fresh air, and it is not wise to stay in such a room. You are killing the cells in your body when you do so, and you will very probably come out of it with a bad cold. When the fresh air strikes you, you feel chilly and you may think you are taking cold then, but in reality you took cold in that room full of foul air.

Ventilation of workshops

Workshops are often poorly ventilated. No person should ever work in a badly ventilated place. The labor unions frequently strike for higher wages, but until recently a strike for better ventilation was rarely heard of. Better ventilation would be practically equal to an increase in wages, because there would be fewer doctors' bills to pay, and less likelihood of losing work through illness. Always have plenty of pure, fresh air wherever you are—in school, in bed, at work, or at play.

Why we should breathe through the nose

The cells in the skin of the nose secrete a watery fluid, and this fluid serves to moisten the air as it passes through the nose. Dry air irritates the mucous membrane which lines the nose, throat, and lungs, and it is very important that the air be moistened before it reaches the throat. Air is also warmed as it passes through the nose. Cold air is irritating to the throat and lungs. The small hairs in the nose catch the dust and dirt in the air and prevent it from going into the lungs.

The nose was made to breathe through, and all the air that goes into your lungs should pass through your nose, in order that it may be moistened, warmed, and cleansed.

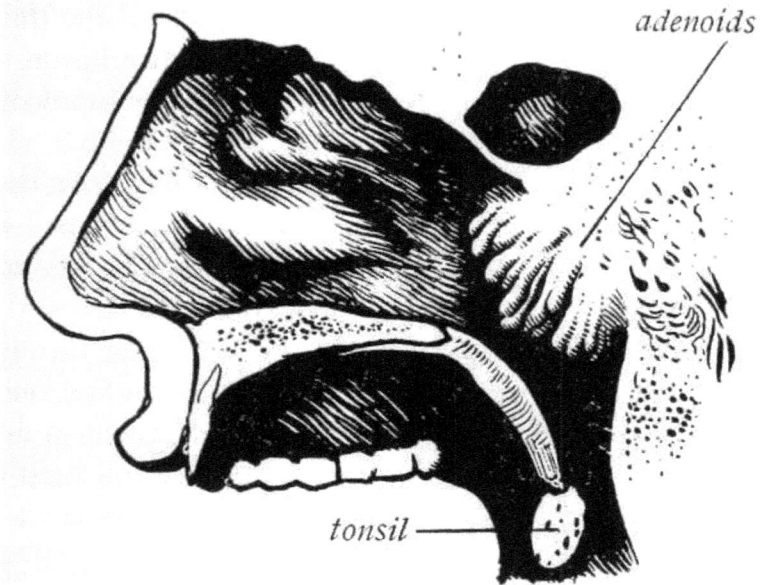

FIG. 28. Showing position of adenoids and tonsils in the throat.

Why some children breathe through the mouth

Frequently we see boys and girls breathing through the mouth. They do this because there is something in the nose that prevents the air from passing freely through it. If there were nothing in the way, the child would breathe through the nose instead of the mouth, because the natural way of breathing is through the nose.

The most common reason for mouth-breathing is the growth of small lumps in the throat just behind the nose. These little lumps are called adenoids. They are not natural, and should be taken out. We do not know why they grow in some children and not in others, but we do know that they should be taken out so that the child can breathe easily through the nose. Large tonsils also cause boys and girls to breathe through the mouth. Tonsils that are large enough to cause the child to breathe through the mouth ought always to be taken out. Large tonsils and adenoids are often found in the same child.

When a child breathes through his mouth all the time, his face takes on a peculiar shape. His upper lip grows long, his lower jaw drops back, and his whole face looks flat. His voice has a peculiar sound, and he finds it very hard to keep up in his classes at school. Children with adenoids and large tonsils are always backward in their school work, and may become deaf if the adenoids and tonsils are not removed.

If you breathe through your mouth instead of through the nose, go to the doctor and let him see if you have adenoids or large tonsils; if you have, let him take them out. You cannot possibly grow into a strong, healthy man or woman if you have adenoids and do not have them removed.

Questions. 1. What does the body take out of the air? 2. What does the body put into the air? 3. What effect does impure air have on the body? 4. Why should one sleep with windows open? 5. What causes the unpleasant odor in a crowded room? 6. How would workmen benefit by properly ventilated workshops? 7. Name the helpful ways in which the air is changed while passing through the nose. 8. Why do some children breathe through the mouth? 9. What effect comes from mouth-breathing?

Remember. 1. Impure air destroys health. 2. Never sleep in a room where the window is closed. 3. Avoid going into public places or workshops that are not well ventilated. 4. Air must pass through the nose before it is fit for the lungs. 5. Mouth-breathing is not natural and is usually due to some defect that can easily be cured.

CHAPTER XII

REST ESSENTIAL TO HEALTH

Why exercise is necessary

Exercise is necessary to make our bodies grow and become strong. If we stayed in bed all the time, our muscles would not grow and we could not even walk. If we did not exercise them, the cells in our brains would not grow and we should not know anything. Every part of our body must have exercise, that is, each part must do some work every day. If we used only one part of the body and did not give the other parts any work to do, only the part that we used would grow, while all the rest of the body would be small and weak.

Proportion of rest required

While every part should do some work each day, the whole body needs also to have a proper amount of rest. Even the heart, which seems to be working all the time, must rest. It rests between each beat. The muscles with which we breathe rest between each breath. Every person must have a certain amount of rest each day. A man should have at least eight hours' sleep in every twenty-four hours; boys and girls should have from nine to ten hours' sleep in every twenty-four. It is only while we are sleeping that we have complete rest.

Effect of overwork

Everybody should have some work to do. Boys and girls should learn that work is a part of life, though they should not be expected to do too much. They should not be required to get up at four o'clock in the morning and work until eight, then go to school until four in the afternoon, and then work again until dark. They cannot do this and keep well. Such children will surely neglect their lessons and will fail to keep up in their classes. It is not the children's fault, but the fault of the people who give them so much to do outside of school.

Sometimes bright children fall behind in their classes and seem to be sleepy during school hours. Very often these children do not have to do any work at home, but play all the time they are out of school. We usually find that these children not only play all the afternoon, but also go to parties at night and often stay up until midnight.

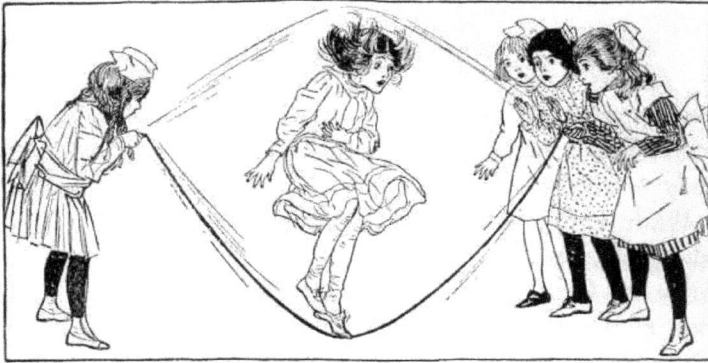

FIG. 29. Children work when they play. The little girl skipping rope is killing the body cells by overwork; she has skipped more than one hundred times and is exhausted.

Ways in which children overwork their bodies

You may think it is not work to go to a party, but it really is. You are working the muscles and the cells of your brain when you are playing games, and these get tired from play work just as they do from working. It is more fun to do play work than to do real work, but the cells are tired and need rest after either kind of exercise. When you go to a party and stay up until midnight, you do not get nine hours of sleep. How do you expect the cells of your bodies to get enough rest when you treat them in this way?

Another thing you do at parties is to eat food that tastes good, but which is not good building material or nourishing for the cells of the body. These things eaten late at night stay in your stomach long after you have gone to bed, and the cells of your stomach do not have a chance to rest at all.

Children should have their parties in the afternoon. You can have just as much fun at a party in the afternoon as you can at night, and then your stomach will have time to dispose of the cake and candies you have eaten, and will be ready to rest when you go to bed.

Small children should be in bed by eight o'clock at night, and even big girls and boys should be asleep by ten o'clock every night. If you do not give your bodies rest, you can never grow into strong men and women.

The importance of regular meals

We have learned that every part of the body needs regular rest. Your stomach is a part of your body. In the stomach and intestines all the food is changed so that the little cells can make use of it. Do you think the cook would serve good meals if she were kept cooking all the time, both night and day? You know she would soon stop cooking for you if you did not give her time to rest. Your stomach does work that is even more important to you than cooking.

Why meals should be at least four hours apart

It takes about four hours for your stomach to dispose of what you give it at a single meal. If you eat your breakfast at eight o'clock, your stomach is going to be kept busy to get rid of it by noon. Of course you expect to give it more work to do at noon; that is, you expect to eat a good luncheon. It will be after four o'clock by the time your stomach has finished the task you put on it at noon, and there will be only about an hour and a half for the stomach to rest before you will be ready to give it another four hours' task, digesting your supper. This means that your stomach cannot go to sleep until ten o'clock. If you eat three meals a day, you will give your stomach just about two hours' rest between eight in the morning and ten at night. If you let it rest from ten at night until eight in the morning, it is not likely to give you any trouble.

When and why candy eating is harmful

Some people will not let their stomachs rest at all. Often boys and girls give their stomachs extra work to do by eating sweetmeats in the middle of the morning while their stomachs are still busy with breakfast. Then, as soon as school is out in the afternoon, they want to eat more cake and candy, and thus take away from the stomach the little rest it has a right to expect before it goes to work on supper. Then suppose they go to a party and eat again about midnight. How much time will the stomach have to rest before breakfast?

When candy eating is not harmful

Now, I have not said that boys and girls must not eat candy; and what is more, I am not going to say any such thing. You may go home and tell your mother that candy is good for girls and boys and that they like it so well they ought to have it—no, not all the time. Here is the part that some of you will not like. Girls and boys ought to have all they want just after eating luncheon or dinner. If you have eaten a hearty meal, it is entirely safe for you to eat candy then; you will not be giving extra work to your stomach, for the candy will be taken care of along with the rest of the meal.

Questions. 1. Why should we all take exercise? 2. How much rest is needed each day? 3. Name some of the effects of overwork. 4. How do children overwork their bodies? 5. Why should children have their parties in the afternoon? 6. Why should meal hours be regular? 7. When and why is candy eating harmful? 8. When is candy eating not harmful?

Remember. 1. Proper rest is necessary to health. 2. Rest from play is as necessary as rest from work. 3. You must give the stomach rest by having regular meal hours and by eating nothing between meals.

CHAPTER XIII

CARE OF THE EYE AND EAR

The loss of sight

Sight is one of the greatest blessings we have. Think how dreadful it is to be blind. If you take care of your eyes, there is no reason why you should be blind; but if you do not take care of your eyes, there is a possibility that you may lose your sight. Most of the blind people in the world became blind because their eyes were not given proper care, and most of this lack of care happened when these people were babies.

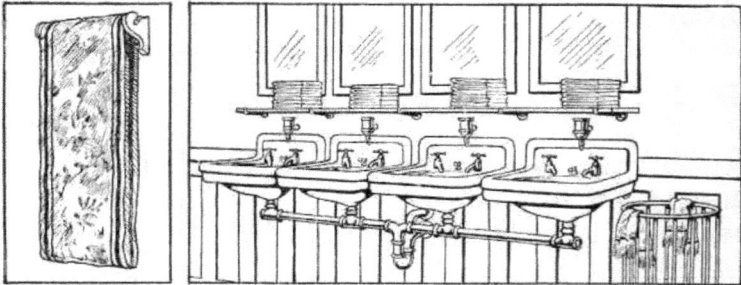

FIGS. 30 and 31. The roller towel is a common source of infection of eyes in schools; every school should have properly constructed wash-rooms, with individual towels.

How germs get into the eyes

Many of the diseases that affect the eyes are catching. They are not carried through the air, but are transmitted by the use of a towel or handkerchief used by someone who had the disease. Never use the towel or handkerchief that another has used.

Germs may be rubbed into the eyes. Keep your hands away from your eyes. Your hands may have disease germs on them, and when you rub your eyes you may put the disease germs into them.

How eyes are overworked

Many boys and girls ruin their eyes by making them do too much work. They do this by reading in a poor light, by reading where the light strikes into the eyes, or by reading in a bad position, as when in bed or lying down. When you are reading, drawing, or doing any work with the eyes, always have the best light possible, which means that the light should fall on your book or work over your left shoulder. If you are only reading, it does not make much difference which shoulder the light comes over, provided it comes from behind. If you are writing or drawing, and the light comes over your right shoulder, it makes the shadow of your hand fall just where you want to see.

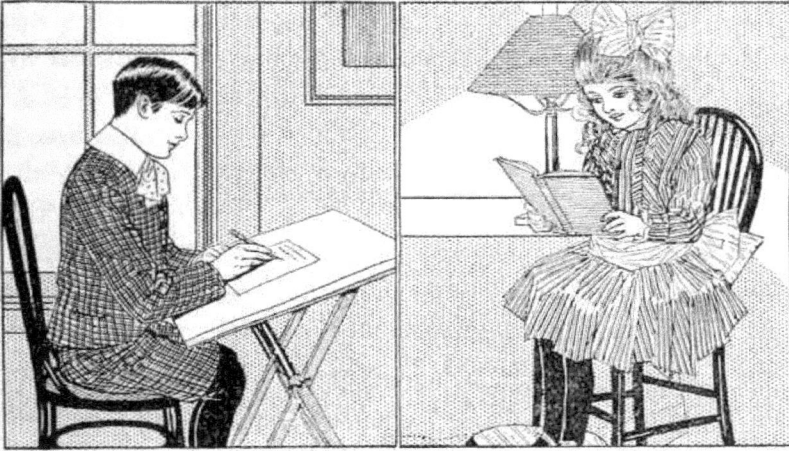

FIGS. 32 and 33. Correct positions for reading and writing.

Another way of working your eyes too much is by trying to see when the eyes are not focused right. Sometimes people are said to be near-sighted, because they cannot see very well at a distance. This is due to the fact that the eyeball is too long, so that the lens does not cause the rays of light to focus on the retina. Some people are called far-sighted. This means that they can see well at a distance, but that it is hard for them to see things close to them. Far-sighted children can usually see things near by, but they do this by making the muscle that rules the lens of the eye work too hard.

Method of testing the eyes

Probably your teacher has a test chart and can tell you whether your eyes are properly focused. If your eyes are not focused right, that is, if you cannot see the line of letters marked **20** when you are twenty feet from this chart, there is something wrong with your eyes. In that case, you are not only injuring them by trying to study, but you are hurting the whole body by overworking a part of it. If you cannot see the letters on the test card clearly at a distance of twenty feet, ask your father to send you to a specialist who will fit you with the proper glasses or will treat your eyes so that you can see well.

How to test the hearing

Sometimes children are backward in their school work because they cannot hear well. Your teacher can test your hearing by holding a watch near your ear. If you cannot hear a watch tick when it is held six feet from your ear, ask your father to take you to your doctor, that he may treat your ears.

How to care for the ears

If your hearing is perfect, the best way to take care of the ears is to let them alone. Never try to dig into the canal that leads to the middle ear. The ears must of course be washed to keep them clean, but in washing the ear you should not touch the delicate canal leading to the drum. A great specialist once said, "Never put anything smaller than your elbow into your ear," to which another great specialist added, "And wrap a towel around your elbow." Never try to dig the wax out of your ears; it belongs in your ears; it is there for a purpose, so let it alone. If it becomes hardened, you cannot get it out and will only injure your ears in trying to do so. An ear spoon is a dangerous thing.

Questions. 1. State the chief cause of loss of sight. 2. How can you keep germs out of your eyes? 3. Name three ways by which you may overwork the eyes. 4. Tell how to take care of the ears.

Remember. 1. Overworking the eyes is as injurious as overworking the stomach. 2. Keep your hands away from your eyes; germs on your hands may get into your eyes and cause them to become sore. 3. You overwork your eyes when you try to read or write in a poor light or in a bad position, as when lying down. 4. You overwork your eyes when you try to study with eyes that are not properly focused. 5. Keep your fingers out of your ears. 6. Take care of your ears by letting them alone.

CHAPTER XIV

CARE OF THE SKIN

If you break or cut the skin on your body, you make an opening through which germs can get in. You cannot always help breaking your skin, but you can always wash the break with soap and water, and put a clean cloth over it to keep out germs.

The work of the sweat glands

The work of the little sweat glands is very important to your health. These glands are just as important as the kidneys, and if they did not do their work, you would die very quickly. If your body is covered with dirt, the work of these glands is seriously interfered with; and when the sweat glands are not doing their full amount of work, the kidneys must do more than their share. It is never right to make one part of your body do the work intended for another part.

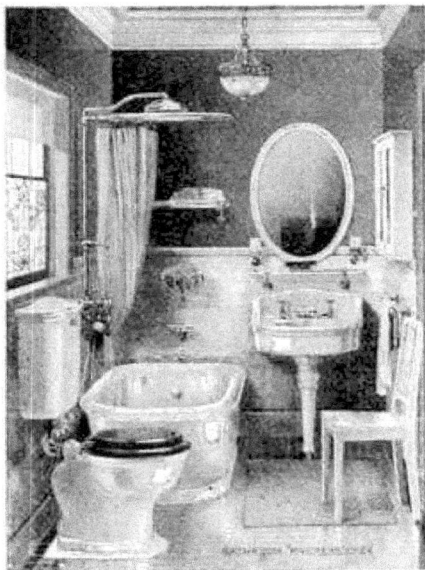

FIG. 34. A model bathroom.

When the body is dirty, not only are the sweat glands interfered with, but the little sebaceous (oil) glands become plugged up, and blackheads appear on the face and body.

Importance of bathing

In order that the various glands of the skin may be kept in good health, it is necessary for us to keep clean. To do this we wash our faces and hands and bathe our bodies. Someone may ask, "How often ought a person to take a bath?" The question cannot be answered, except to say, "Just as often as may be necessary for you to keep absolutely clean." Some people do not have to bathe as often as others, but no one can keep clean unless he takes a bath at least twice a week.

Hot or cold baths

Another question that is frequently asked is, "Is it better to take a bath in cold or hot water?" This is another question that cannot be answered in the same way for every person. A cold bath is more stimulating than a warm bath. If, after you have taken a cold bath and rubbed yourself briskly with a rough towel, the skin becomes red and warm, a cold bath is best for you. But if, after you have taken a cold bath and rubbed yourself for not more than ten minutes, the skin appears bluish and cold, a cold bath is not good for you, and you should not take it. A cold bath should always be taken in the morning, just after getting out of bed, and a warm bath should always be taken in the evening, just before going to bed.

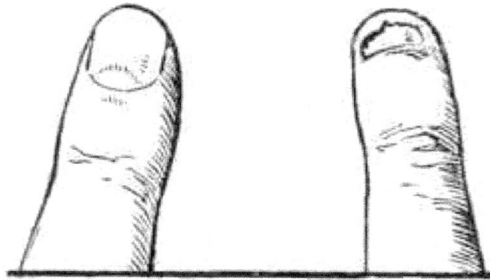

FIG. 35. A nail properly cared for, and a nail not properly cared for. Which should you prefer to have?

How to care for the nails

The finger nails and toe nails are a part of the skin and they also need to be taken care of. You will see at the root of your finger nails a thin layer of skin that is inclined to grow out with the nail. If this skin is not kept pushed back it becomes rough, breaks into little shreds, and forms "hang nails." This little band of skin should always be kept carefully pushed back. The finger nails should be kept evenly and neatly trimmed, but they should not be cut so close to the skin that the ends of the fingers project beyond the nails. The nails are for the protection of the ends of the fingers and toes. Nails that are trimmed unevenly and nails that are bitten off are ugly and indicate untidy habits. The shape of the nails should follow the outline of the ends of the finger. Neither is it a sensible fashion to trim the nails to points or to let them grow very long.

The toe nails need attention just as much as do the finger nails. They should be trimmed to follow the shape of the toe. Failure to trim the toe nails properly will result in ingrowing nails.

Dirt is very likely to collect under the nails. This should always be carefully cleaned out. You cannot wash this dirt out unless you use a stiff nail brush. If you clean your nails just after you wash your hands, you will find that it will be much easier to get the dirt out while the dirt and the nail are both softened by the soap and water. In cleaning your nails, use a dull nail cleaner or a smooth wooden stick. Do not scrape the inside of the nail with a sharp knife. This scraping of the inside of the nails will cause them to catch the dirt more easily, as well as to grow thicker and thicker until they become very ugly. Neat, clean finger nails help to make pretty hands; dirty, untidy nails spoil the prettiest hands.

Questions. 1. What are the uses of the sweat glands? 2. How often should people take baths? 3. How can you tell whether a hot or a cold bath is better for you? 4. Tell how finger nails should be cared for. 5. How should toe nails be treated?

Remember. 1. If you do not keep your body clean, the glands of the skin cannot do their work properly. 2. Every person should take a bath at least twice a week; some persons need a bath every day in order to keep clean. 3. If you take a bath in cold water, and the skin does not become warm and pink when you rub it with a rough towel, a cold bath is not good for you. 4. Cold baths should be taken in the morning on getting up. 5. Warm baths should be taken in the evening before going to bed. 6. Finger nails should always be kept clean and neat; dirty, untidy nails make ugly hands.

CHAPTER XV

COMMON POISONS TO BE AVOIDED

Many people are killing the cells of their bodies by taking certain poisons into them. There are many kinds of poisons that can be taken into the body, but we are going to learn now about only two. These are tobacco and alcohol.

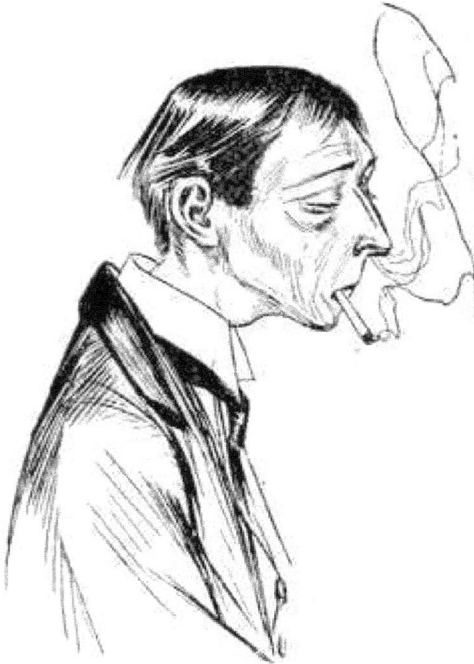

FIG. 36. Effect of cigarette smoking.

Proof that tobacco is a poison

Tobacco is a poison. Those of you who have tried to smoke know this, because it made you sick the first time you tried it. There are many other indications that tobacco is a poison. We know that it affects the red blood cells in such a way that they do not carry the oxygen as well as do those of people who do not smoke. We know that it has a very bad effect on the heart and that it interferes with the action of the nervous system.

The extra work caused by tobacco

When certain poisons get into the body, the blood makes something that will counteract the effects of those poisons. After one has used tobacco for some time, the cells of the body will take care of the tobacco poison by making an antidote for it. More than this, they begin to want it all the time. The tobacco user forces the cells of his body to make an antidote for this poison every time he uses tobacco. Thus he makes the cells do work that is unnecessary, and keeps them from doing work that is necessary.

Other bad effects of tobacco: (1) On the nose and throat

Tobacco smoke irritates the cells that line the throat and nose and causes inflammation. This is why so many smokers have catarrh. Smoking is not the only cause of catarrh, for people who do not smoke often have this trouble, but it is one of the most frequent causes. Smoking also irritates the throat so badly that many of those who smoke have "smoker's throat." This is a bad form of sore throat that can be cured only by stopping the use of tobacco.

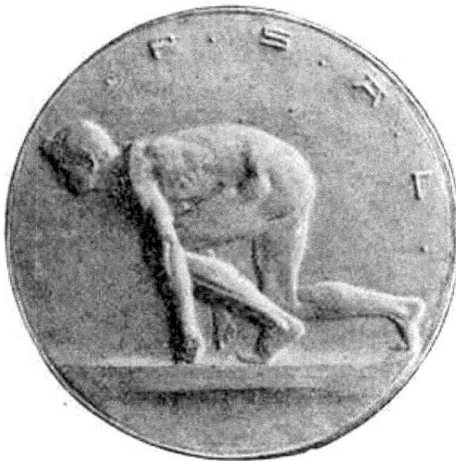

FIG. 37. The athlete knows that alcohol and tobacco are foes to speed, strength, and nervous control. (*From photograph of "The Sprinter," modelled by Dr. R. Tait McKenzie.*)

(2) On the blood

People who smoke a great deal have fewer red corpuscles (the little red cells of the blood) than those who do not smoke. Especially is this true of cigarette smokers. It is the lack of red blood cells that causes the cigarette smoker to look pale and sallow.

It is probably not the direct effect of tobacco that causes the loss of red blood cells, but something that is connected with the act of smoking. When you take smoke into your mouth, you take in at the same time a gas known as *carbon monoxid.* This gas is very poisonous to the body, and combines with the red blood cells in such a way that they cannot take up the oxygen in the lungs and carry it to the rest of the cells in the body. The cigarette smoker almost always inhales the smoke, and thus he absorbs a great deal more of the carbon monoxid than the man who does not inhale the smoke. Of course, the more of this gas he takes into his body, the more red blood cells will be affected and the less oxygen will be taken to the other cells.

(3) On the nervous system

We do not know just how tobacco affects the cells of the nervous system. It may be that they are affected mostly by being deprived of oxygen, or it may be that the tobacco affects them directly. However the harm is done, we know that the cells of the nervous system are affected by tobacco. One of the nerves that is most commonly affected by the use of tobacco is the nerve of the eye, the nerve that enables us to see. We know that when people use tobacco a great deal they sometimes lose their sight. This does not happen to everyone who uses tobacco, but you can never tell whom it will affect in this way. The only safe thing to do is not to use tobacco, and then you will know that you will not lose your sight from this cause.

(4) On the stomach

The use of tobacco affects the stomach. People who use tobacco a great deal are likely to have indigestion. The tobacco causes this probably by depriving the stomach cells of oxygen through its effect on the blood cells.

(5) On the heart

Tobacco has a very bad effect on the heart. People who use much tobacco have what they call "palpitation of the heart," but doctors call it "tobacco heart," because it is caused by the use of tobacco. No insurance company will insure a person who has "tobacco heart."

Most boys grow up to be men before they manage to use enough tobacco to cause tobacco heart. However, long before they are grown, they show that the tobacco has affected their hearts, because they are short of breath and stand about as much chance of winning a race as does a mouth-breather.

Effects of alcohol:

The effect of alcohol is a subject on which I want to speak very plainly and frankly, because I do not want the boys and girls who read this to get the same idea that I got when I was in school, or to be affected by it as I was. When I was a little boy I was taught that if a person drank alcohol in any form the lining of his stomach would be eaten up. In proof of this statement I was shown a picture of an ulcerated stomach that was said to have resulted from drinking whisky. Naturally I expected to find that people who drank whisky would not be able to eat anything at all, or would be troubled a great deal with pain in their stomachs. To my surprise, I found that many people had ulcers of the stomach who never took an alcoholic drink, while many of those who drank a great deal seemed to have the best of appetites and were never troubled with their stomachs. As a result, I came to the conclusion that all this talk about the evil effects of alcohol was foolishness. Later I studied medicine, and learned that the effect of alcohol on the stomach is, in reality, the least of its evils. But I want to impress upon you that, as a result of forty years' study, I consider alcohol the most dangerous thing in the world to-day. By "alcohol" we mean any drink that contains alcohol, such as whisky, wine, brandy, beer, etc.

(1) On the stomach

When alcohol is taken into the stomach, it first causes a congestion; that is, it causes an increase in the quantity of blood in the blood vessels of the stomach. It might seem that this would aid digestion in the stomach, but it does not, because alcohol affects the food in the stomach in such a way that it prevents the gastric juice from acting on the food. If the use of alcohol is persisted in, it causes the little cells in the stomach that make the gastric juice to become filled with fat, and then those cells cannot make the gastric juice. Thus, continued use of alcohol causes a smaller supply of gastric juice, and the food passes from the stomach into the intestines without having been acted upon by the gastric juice, as it should have been. The result is that the food decomposes in the intestines and a poison is formed. This poison is taken up by the vessels that carry the food from the intestines and kills a great many of the cells of the body.

Alcohol does not burn holes in the stomach, but it destroys the usefulness of the stomach by its action on the cells that secrete the gastric juice.

(2) On the liver

When alcohol is taken into the stomach, very little of it reaches the intestines. It is rapidly absorbed by the lining of the stomach and passes into the blood. The blood from the stomach goes directly to the liver. The alcohol makes the cells of the liver hard and causes them to become filled with fat, as it does the cells of the stomach. In this way it destroys the action of these cells and prevents their doing the work for which they are intended. From the liver the alcohol goes with the blood to all parts of the body, and it has its influence on all the cells in the body. This influence is always harmful.

(3) On the body's powers of resistance

We know that when a man who is in the habit of drinking gets pneumonia, he is far more likely to die than is one who is not in the habit of using alcoholic drinks. The man who drinks cannot resist the effects of disease as can one who does not drink. This shows that the use of alcohol reduces our resisting powers, and puts our cells in such condition that we cannot overcome the effects of disease.

People who are sick with a slow disease like consumption are often advised by their friends to take whisky to brace them up. It is true that the immediate effect of the whisky is to make the patient feel a little better, but the final effect is to leave him in a much weaker condition than before. More than this, the cells are much less able to resist the disease germs than they were before the alcohol was taken. When people are exposed to such diseases as scarlet fever and smallpox, they may think that if they take a drink of whisky they will not be so liable to contract the disease. It is just the other way. The alcohol reduces the resisting powers of the cells of the body, and anything that does this renders a person more liable to contract any disease to which he is exposed.

(4) On the nervous system

The effect of alcohol on the cells of the nervous system is very marked. Continued use will injure the nervous system and result in a kind of insanity called delirium tremens. It will also cause other forms of insanity. The effect of alcohol on the parent is passed on to the children of the next generation, and even beyond this. A large percentage of idiotic children are the offspring of alcoholic parents.

(5) On the morals

The use of alcohol numbs the sense of right and wrong. More young men have become criminals from the use of alcohol than from any other one cause. Anyone who reads the daily papers can see that many criminals give the use of alcohol as an excuse for having committed a crime.

(6) On brain work

Some people will tell you that alcohol stimulates the brain, so that one can work faster and better. This is not true. Tests have been made in this matter, and it has been found that men doing mental work will work about one tenth slower and make one fourth more mistakes when given one drink of whisky a day, than they will when not given any whisky. If *one* drink of whisky a day thus reduces a man's power and accuracy in doing mental work, what do you think three drinks, or ten drinks will do?

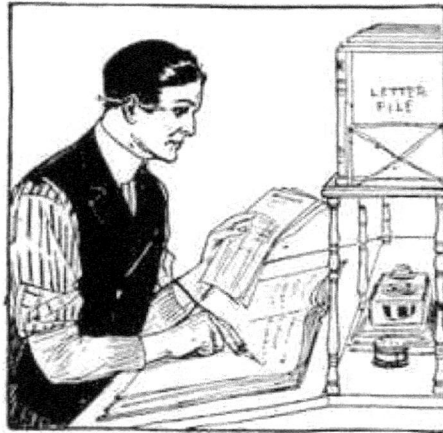

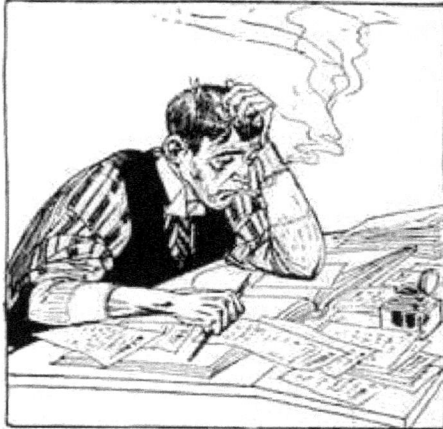

FIG. 38. The mind not clouded by alcohol works quickly and makes few mistakes.

FIG. 39. The mind clouded by alcohol works slowly and makes many mistakes.

What business men think of men who drink

Many business men drink, and they know the results of alcohol not only from the effects they have observed in others, but also from the effect they know it to have on themselves. When a man applies to them for a position, these business men almost invariably ask him if he drinks. The man who does not drink stands nine chances in ten of securing the position, while the man who drinks stands only one chance in ten. This shows what business men think of the effect of alcohol, even when taken in moderate quantities. They know that it reduces a man's power to do mental as well as physical work, that it causes him to make mistakes, and that it may finally destroy his morals and result in his becoming a thief or a criminal.

Questions. 1. How do we know that tobacco is a poison? 2. How does tobacco make extra work for the body? 3. What effect does tobacco have on the nose and throat? 4. What is the effect of tobacco on the blood? 5. On the nervous system? 6. On the heart? 7. Mention some of the false ideas about the effect of alcohol. 8. How does alcohol affect the stomach? 9. The liver? 10. In what ways does alcohol reduce the resisting powers of the body? 11. How does alcohol affect the nervous system? 12. How does it influence mental work? 13. What do business men think of drinkers? 14. What influence has alcohol on the next generation?

Remember. 1. Tobacco is a poison that has a very bad effect on the nervous system, the blood, the heart, the stomach, the nose, and the throat. 2. Alcohol is a poison and not a food. 3. Alcohol injures the stomach, the liver, and the nervous system. 4. Alcohol reduces the power to do accurate mental work. 5. Alcohol numbs the sense of right and wrong, and encourages crime.

PART II
THE ENEMIES OF HEALTH

CHAPTER XVI

DISEASE GERMS

We have learned that the body is made up of cells, and that each cell is alive. The cells in our bodies cannot live separately. There are, however, certain animals and plants that are each made up of a single cell. These animals and plants are called germs, and some of them cause disease.

Different germs cause different diseases

These germs are so exceedingly small that we can see them only with the aid of a microscope. They differ in appearance one from another, as a pine tree differs from an ash, or an American child from a Chinese child. When you plant your garden, you put sweet peas in one place and asters in another, and you know that you will have sweet peas growing where you planted the pea seeds, and asters growing where the aster seeds were put. So it is with these little germs; you will no more get tuberculosis from typhoid fever germs than you would get asters from pea seeds.

Now, while there are many, many kinds of germs in the world, there are only certain ones that cause certain diseases, and we have learned where these germs like to live and how to kill them. We also know that they come only from some person or animal sick with the particular disease which they cause. Typhoid fever germs are not given off by a person suffering with tuberculosis, nor are diphtheria germs given off by a typhoid fever patient, but the germ of each disease is given off by some person or animal suffering from that particular disease.

How sickness due to germs can be prevented

If we kill all the germs that come from people sick with a certain disease, no one else can catch that disease. Knowing this, it seems unnecessary for anyone ever to be sick with disease that is caused by a germ. This is literally true, and the only reason that we have germ diseases is because we do not kill the germs that come from the sick people.

Professor Irving Fisher of Yale University has said, "It is entirely possible to wipe out consumption within a single generation." It may not actually be done so quickly, but it is certain that the disease can finally be wiped out, though it may require many generations to accomplish it.

Why, then, are germ diseases allowed to exist? Simply because so many people do not know the facts; and because many who do know will not take the trouble to kill the germs, even when they realize that some one else may get the disease as a result of their carelessness. What do you think of a woman who said, "I do not care if my neighbor's children do get scarlet fever from us; she is not a friend of mine, any way"? A woman has been heard to make such a statement to a health officer. It is just such people as this who spread disease.

Questions. 1. How may germs be compared to seeds? 2. What do we know about disease germs that will help us to get rid of them? 3. How is it possible for us to get rid of consumption and other germ diseases?

Remember. 1. While there are many kinds of germs in the world, only a few cause disease. 2. The germ that causes a certain disease will cause that disease and no other. 3. It is entirely possible to kill all the germs that cause disease.

CHAPTER XVII

ENCOURAGEMENT OF DISEASE BY UNCLEANLY HABITS

We shall not try to learn here all the ways by which it is possible to destroy the germs of disease as they come from sick people. But there are certain rules (we sometimes call them fundamental principles) that you must know, if you hope to keep well and to prevent others from getting sick.

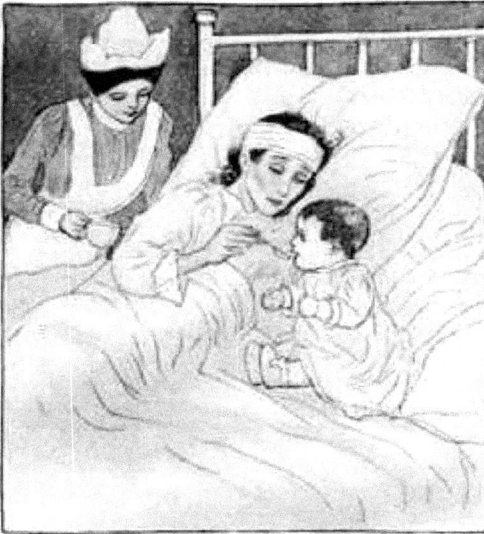

FIG. 40. How diseases are frequently transmitted to children.

Why we should stay away from the sickroom

The first of these rules is: *Do not go into the room where any one is sick unless it is absolutely necessary.* No one but the nurse should sleep in the room with a sick person. We know that certain diseases are communicable (catching), but it has not yet been determined whether some others are communicable or not. It has not been proved, for instance, that we cannot catch rheumatism from another person. Only a few years ago it was believed that one could not take consumption from another person, but now we know that this is the very way to get it. Therefore, stay away from sick people as much as possible. It is not good for the patient to have people around him, and it is dangerous for the well to come in contact with the sick.

Not using things used by the sick

The second rule is: *Do not use anything used by a sick person until it has been washed.* This is a good rule to apply to things used by a well person also. It is neither safe nor pleasant to eat from the spoon or fork, or to use the napkin or towel which has been used by someone else.

Sometimes children think the food prepared for a sick person is ever so much nicer than that set before themselves, and wish they could have a little of it. How often have we seen a sick mother give her little ones "a taste" from the spoon with which she is eating. This is very dangerous, and if she knew it, the mother would cut her hand off before exposing her children to this danger.

Reason for scalding things used by the sick

Third: *Everything taken from a sickroom should be boiled before it is used again.* The knives, forks, and plates should not be put with other dishes until after they have been separately washed and boiled. Towels, napkins, bedding, and clothing from a sickroom should not be washed with other bedding and clothing, but should be washed and boiled separately. Some people send out the clothes from the sickroom with the rest of their washing, and in this way give disease to others.

How excreta from the sick should be treated

Fourth: *All discharges (sputum, urine, bowel discharges, and matter from sores) from any sick person should be thoroughly disinfected before being finally disposed of.* The sputum should be received on little rags or paper napkins, and burned; and the other discharges should be disinfected with some poison that will kill the germs. We shall say more about disinfection when we come to study the prevention of special diseases.

Necessity of washing the hands after touching the sick

Fifth: *Every person who touches a sick person, or handles anything that comes from a sickroom, should immediately wash his hands.* Unless he washes his hands at once, the germs which may be on them may get into his mouth.

Sixth: *Dirt, which is an indirect cause of disease, must not be allowed to accumulate.* If your yard were full of dirt, garbage, and manure, it would not cause disease unless the germs of some disease became planted there. But such a place is an indirect cause of disease, in that it furnishes a fine place for germs to grow in. If a fly with typhoid germs on its feet were to alight in such a yard, the germs would be planted in a most favorable spot and would grow very fast.

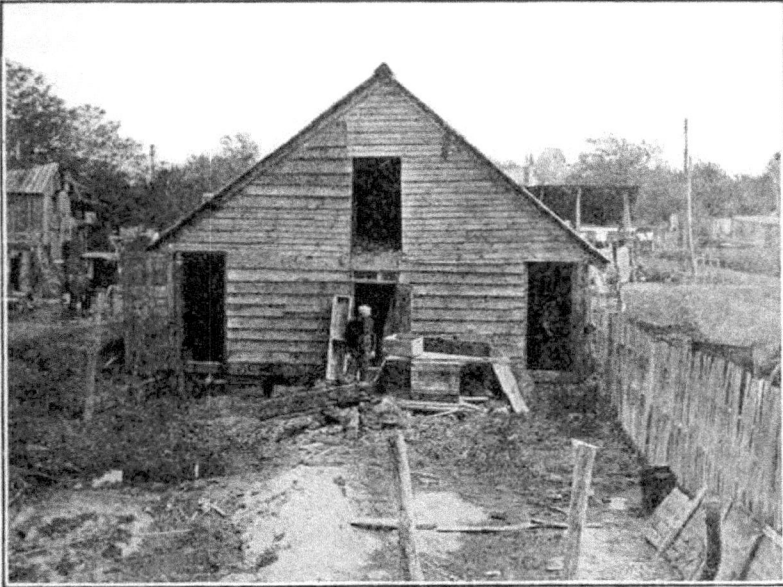

FIG. 41. A place that is an indirect cause of disease, since it furnishes a fine place for germs to grow in.

None of the disease germs like sunshine; neither do they like dry places. They die very quickly in the sunlight, and grow very slowly, if at all, in dry places; but in damp, dark places they grow very fast. Dirty back yards make ideal gardens for germs.

Let a fly with germs on its feet alight in a clean yard where sunshine can reach every corner, and what chance will the germs have to grow? They will not even get a start. Hence, while disease cannot be caused by dirt, disease germs stand a very good chance of living where there is plenty of dirt and no sunshine. Filthy habits are on an equality with filthy conditions, and go hand in hand with them. One of the worst of habits, and a cause of much sickness, is that of answering Nature's calls in places other than the closet.

Questions. 1. Why should you never make unnecessary visits to a sick person? 2. Why should you avoid anything used by a sick person? 3. Why should everything taken from a sickroom be scalded? 4. What should be done with all discharges from a sick person? 5. How is dirt a source of disease?

Remember. 1. Unless it is necessary, do not go into a room where anyone is sick. 2. Never sleep in a room with a sick person. 3. Never eat from a spoon or plate that has been used by another. 4. Boil all the articles taken from the room of a sick person. 5. Always wash your hands after touching a sick person or anything that comes from his room. 6. Sunshine kills germs; let the sunshine into every corner of your house.

CHAPTER XVIII

FLIES AS CARRIERS OF DISEASE

How germs get into our bodies

Disease germs get into our bodies in three principal ways: they are eaten with our food; they are taken in with the air we breathe; and they get in through breaks in our skin, even though these breaks be very small, as when made by the bite of a mosquito or other insect.

How germs get into our food:

(1) From the air

How do germs get into our food or drink? You must remember that these germs are extremely small, so small that many of them can be carried by a particle of dust that you can see only in a ray of sunshine. When the germs become dried, they float about on these particles of dust, the dust alights on our food, which is moist and warm, and the germs immediately begin to grow.

(2) From the hands

Another way by which germs get on food is from the hands through which it passes. Did you ever think how many people handle an apple? First, the man who picks it from the tree; then the examiner in the packing house where apples are taken to see that they are the right kind to be packed in a certain box. Then it is wiped off by a boy or girl—handling number three; then it is wrapped in paper—number four. Next it is packed in a box, but in this case the paper protects the apple from dirty hands. When the merchant buys the apples he feels several of them, and puts them out on the display shelf; this makes handling number five. Everyone who thinks of buying apples will touch one or more of them, and when they are sold the clerk handles them again. In other words, every apple goes through the hands of at least seven people before you get it. Do you not think it needs washing?

Go into a butcher shop and see how many people will put their dirty fingers on the meat. Some of them even keep their gloves on when they do this. Imagine how many germs may be planted on the finger of a glove.

Our whole method of displaying foods for sale is wrong. The customer can see the fruits, vegetables, and meats just as well in a glass case as when they are on an open counter or shelf, and nothing is gained by poking a dirty finger into a piece of beef, or by rubbing your hands over the apples. A glass case not only will protect the fruits and meats from such practices, but will keep out germ-laden dust and flies whose feet are covered with germs.

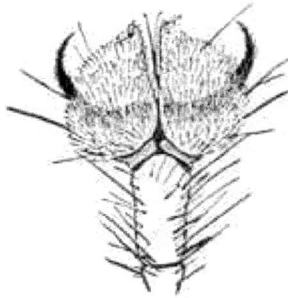

FIG. 42. The foot of a fly, highly magnified.

(3) From flies

Probably the most common source of germs on food is the fly. Did you ever watch a fly very closely for a long time? Did you ever happen to see a manure pile early in the morning and notice how many tiny flies are on it? These flies have just been hatched.

Breeding places of flies

Flies like manure because it is the best place they can find in which to lay their eggs. Each female fly lays about three hundred eggs. They do not hatch directly into flies, as hen's eggs hatch into chickens, but when the fly's eggs hatch you find maggots, and these maggots later hatch into flies.

The journey of the fly

Turn over the manure some spring morning, and you will see it full of white specks. These specks are maggots that will hatch into flies. Watch the flies as they leave the manure pile and see where they go. If there is a dead dog or cat or a filthy garbage can near, they will fly to it. Then they will go into the water-closet and crawl over the filth there. Their next trip will probably bring them to the kitchen, where they will crawl over the food. From here they will go to the cuspidor and take a drink of water, and will get their feet covered with the dirt that is in the cuspidor. Next they will try a walk over the nipple of the baby's bottle, or they will light on your face, or get into the butter or milk.

After the fly has been in dirty places, he "washes" his face and hands, that is, he rubs his feet together and then rubs them over his head. Did you ever see a fly wash himself with water? No, you never did.

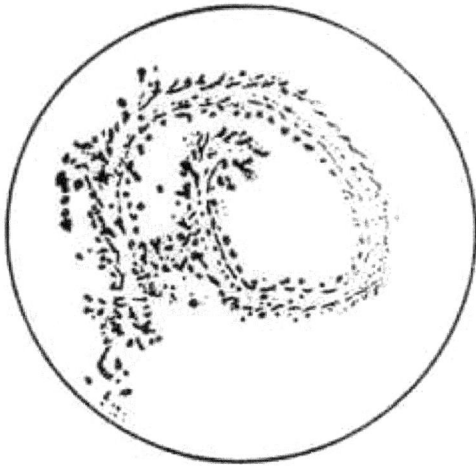

FIG. 43. Where a fly has walked; each little spot represents a growth of germs left by the fly.

After a fly has made his journey, you would suppose that his feet would be covered with dirt and germs, and so they are. Not only does he carry germs on his feet and body but he also eats dirty and diseased things. Moreover, fly specks contain the germs of disease, and the fly is not at all particular about where he puts his specks.

Proof that the fly is a germ carrier

If you let a fly walk over a culture plate, there will be a growth of germs wherever his feet touch. A culture plate is simply a glass plate covered with gelatine or something else in which these germs like to grow, and where they can easily be seen. Each germ will multiply so fast that there will soon be a spot of them large enough to be seen readily with the naked eye. In the picture showing a culture plate over which a fly has walked (Fig. 43), the little specks are not single germs, but each speck represents a growth containing many thousands of germs.

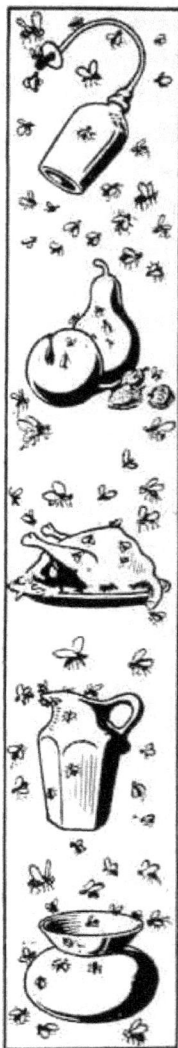

FIG. 44. Flies go from filth to food.

How to get rid of the fly:

How are we going to get rid of flies? We cannot get rid of them entirely, but there are a great many ways by which we can prevent there being so many of them, and whereby we may keep them out of our houses and away from our food.

(1) By removal of manure

We have learned that flies are always found about horse manure, because it makes a good place in which to hatch their eggs. If we could dispose of the manure, there would be one place less for the fly to lay her eggs. Behind barns we usually find piles of manure. It is in these heaps that the fly lays her eggs, not in the little lumps found in the streets. Now, there is no sense in keeping this great pile of manure about any barn. In towns the manure can be put into a box with a cover, so that the flies cannot get at it. In the country every well-managed farm has the barns cleaned out every day, and it would not be much more trouble for the farmer to throw the manure into a wagon and take it to the fields with him, than it is to pile it up beside his barn. If he did this, he would find that there would be few flies about his house.

(2) By covering garbage cans

Even if we were to take every particle of manure away as fast as possible, we should still have some flies, for when flies do not find manure for their hatching places, they will take the next best thing. It must be something dirty; clean things will not answer at all for a fly's home. Next to the manure pile, the fly likes a dirty garbage can, a dead animal, or anything that is decomposing. If she cannot find anything better, she will take a rotting apple; but she does not really like this, and if she cannot find anything better than an old apple in your yard, she will probably go elsewhere to lay her eggs.

(3) By keeping clean yards

We cannot entirely stop the hatching of flies, but if we do away with the old manure piles, keep fresh manure and garbage cans covered, and keep our yards free from everything that can decompose, we shall have very few flies about our houses.

How to keep flies out of the house

Since we cannot get rid of all the flies, the next best thing is to keep the few that may be left out of our houses and away from our food. This we can do by means of wire screens and netting. Wire screens are very cheap, and if there are no wire screens on your house, you should persuade your father to buy some. But a screen will not keep flies out unless it is kept closed, so do your part by never leaving the screen door open for a second longer than is necessary for you to go in or out.

Our houses are not the only places that need screens. Slaughterhouses, butcher shops, candy stores, grocery stores—every place where any kind of food is handled or sold—should be screened. Flies should never be allowed to alight on anything which is to be eaten.

Questions. 1. Name three ways by which germs get into our bodies. 2. How do germs get into our food? 3. Why should foods be screened? 4. Trace the fly from his birth-place to our food. 5. How do we know that flies have germs on their feet? 6. Tell how we can get rid of most of the flies. 7. How can we keep flies out of the house? 8. What can boys and girls do to help keep them out?

Remember. 1. Always wash an apple, pear, or any other fruit before you eat it. 2. All foods are handled by many people, and are not clean until they have been washed. 3. Flies like to live in dirty places, and their feet and legs are covered with germs; get rid of the flies. 4. Flies hatch in manure piles and other dirty places; keep your yard and lot clean so that flies will have no place to lay their eggs. 5. Put screens on the house to keep flies out, and keep the screens closed.

CHAPTER XIX

HOW DISEASE GERMS GET INTO WATER

The water that we drink frequently contains disease germs. It is not always the clearest water that is freest from disease germs, for the germs do not make the water cloudy.

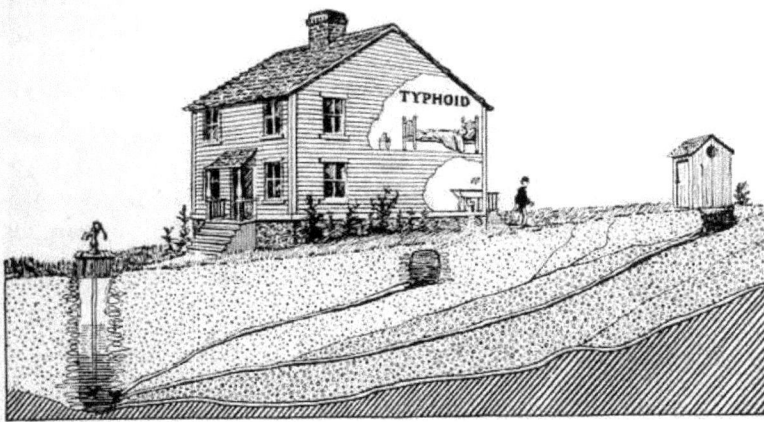

FIG. 45. An improperly located well; notice lines of seepage.

Why sewage should not be put into streams

Water does not get disease germs from the ground, but from man. Almost every town has a sewer system that empties into some stream. This practice was started a long time ago when men thought that running water would purify itself in the course of a few miles. We have learned, however, that this is not true. Germs will continue to live in running water just as they do in any other water, and disease germs will live in a stream from twenty-five to thirty-five days. Estimate how far a stream will flow in that length of time, and you will know how far disease germs will travel in that way. No sewage should ever be allowed to get into a stream until the germs in the sewage have been killed.

Other sources of germs in streams

Sewage is not the only means by which disease germs are carried into streams. Often we find people building barns, slaughterhouses, and mills on the banks of a stream. The filth from barns and slaughterhouses always contains disease germs, and often the filth of mills contains poisons that are just as harmful as germs when taken into our bodies. None of these things should ever be allowed to get into a stream. Water is a very important article of food, and we should take every care to keep it pure.

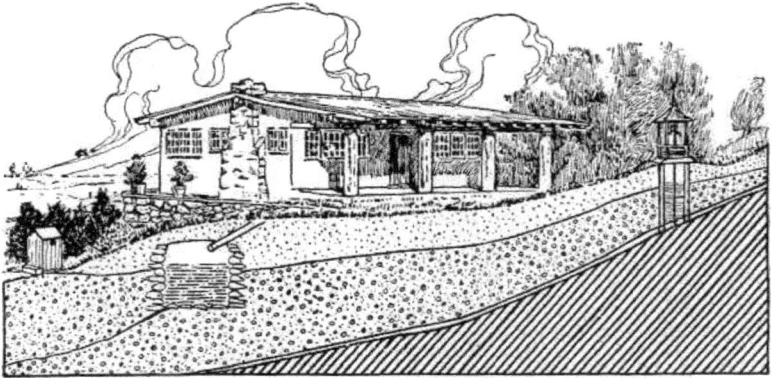

FIG. 46. A properly located well.

How germs get into wells

The water from most wells is clear and cool, but nevertheless may contain many disease germs. "How does this happen?" you ask. Because the well is too close to an out-house or some other source of filth. When a man in the country or in a small town builds a house, he immediately thinks of digging a well just as close to the house as he can, so that he need not carry the water far. Next he thinks of locating the closet, and this, too, he wants near the house. The well and the closet are often near each other, and often the closet is on higher ground than the well. The vault under the closet is seldom water-tight. In fact, the intention of the owner is that a great part of the vault contents shall soak away.

In many localities the ground is an open gravel, and the vault contents run through this gravel into the well, carrying disease germs with them. In one little town, with wells as a source of drinking water, the health officers found that the closet of every house was draining directly into its well. In some countries vaults can be used; but in any region where there is a gravel subsoil, the contents of the closet will find their way into the well, unless the closet is lower than the bottom of the well. In such places the vault must be made water-tight, in order to keep the vault contents out of the well.

Why springs are not always pure

Springs are usually sources of pure water, but do not think that every particle of water that oozes from the ground is a spring. Near a certain town is a so-called "very fine spring." This "spring" appeared after a man had made a cesspool on the hill above, and is simply the drainage from the cesspool. Springs that come from deep sources, however, nearly always contain pure water.

The safest sources of water

The safest source of water for domestic use is a stream that is known to be free from contamination, or a well so deep in the ground that it is hard for any polluting matter to reach it. But remember that sewage may follow a well pipe along the outside and thus reach even a deep well, if the well is not properly protected at the top.

Keep disease germs out of your drinking water. You cannot drown them out and you cannot strain them out, so do not let them get in, for you cannot drink water containing disease germs without running the risk of becoming sick.

Questions. 1. Mention more than one way in which germs get into streams. 2. How long may disease germs live in running water? 3. Mention some instances showing that running water does not purify itself. 4. How do disease germs get into milk? 5. Describe the proper location of a well in regard to refuse. 6. How may springs become polluted? 7. What are the best sources of water for domestic use?

Remember. 1. Disease germs get into water from dirty places along the banks of the streams; they do not come from the ground. 2. Clear water is not always pure; germs do not make the water cloudy or muddy. 3. Wells often become infected by matter from closets seeping into them; make your closet water-tight. 4. Spring water is usually pure, but not all water that oozes out of the ground is spring water.

CHAPTER XX

TRANSMISSION OF DISEASE
THROUGH THE AIR

Disease germs in the air

We take germs into our bodies with the air that we breathe. Since we cannot stop breathing and live, we must see to it that the air we breathe is kept pure.

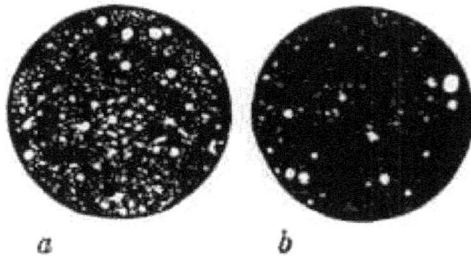

FIG. 47. (a) Prevalence of germs in air of thickly populated districts. (b) Prevalence of germs in air of sparsely populated districts.

There are always more germs in the air of places in which people live closely crowded together than where there are only a few people. This is proved by Figure 47, which shows that many more germs were found on a culture plate exposed in the downtown part of New York City than on another plate exposed far uptown, where there are not so many people. Remember, however, that all germs are not disease germs.

How we may keep disease germs out of the air:

How do the disease germs get into the air? When one sneezes, a spray of droplets is thrown into the air. If the person sneezing has the grip, these droplets contain the germs that cause grip. Whenever a person with consumption coughs, he sprays droplets which contain the germs that cause consumption.

(1) When coughing or sneezing

If a person would hold a handkerchief before his mouth when he coughs or sneezes, these droplets of moisture would not be sprayed into the air, and the disease germs in them would not be scattered about. You ask, "Shall everyone who is sick hold a handkerchief before the mouth when sneezing or coughing?" Everyone, whether sick or well, ought to hold a handkerchief before the mouth when sneezing or coughing. Learn to do this at once, and never forget it.

(2) When spitting

Another way by which disease germs get into the air is from the sputum. People spit on the floor or the sidewalk, and the sputum becomes dried; it is then blown about as dust. The germs of disease are not killed by drying, and when they get into our bodies with the dust which we breathe in, they immediately begin to grow. Disease germs get into the air chiefly through careless habits of coughing, sneezing, and spitting, and these careless habits can easily be prevented.

Why well people should not spit on floor or sidewalk

A boy once said that if he saw a consumptive spit on the sidewalk, he would want to hit him, and to emphasize his remarks he spat on the floor of the room, just as you have seen boys spit on the ground when they were thinking of fighting. There might have been some germs of consumption in the sputum this boy left on the floor. Of course he was very positive that he did not have consumption, but this was no proof that his sputum was free from the germs of this disease.

Remember that it is not only the sick who should never spit on the floor or sidewalk, but that no person should ever spit on any floor or sidewalk, or into any place except into a cuspidor, handkerchief, or spit-cup of some kind. If you spit into a handkerchief, a paper napkin, or a bit of cloth, be sure to burn it as soon as you can, before it becomes dry.

Questions. 1. In what places do we find germs most abundant in the air? 2. How do well-bred people avoid putting disease germs into the air? 3. Why is it important for well people to take the same precautions as sick people?

Remember. 1. Every person should hold a handkerchief before the face when coughing or sneezing. 2. Never spit except into a cuspidor, handkerchief, spit-cup, or other special receptacle. 3. If well people will practice clean habits, the sick will be helped and encouraged to follow their example. 4. Remember: No spit, no consumption.

CHAPTER XXI

INSECTS AS CARRIERS OF DISEASE

Some insects that carry disease

Certain diseases are given to human beings by the bites of insects. We know that certain ticks and mosquitoes carry certain germs. It is also probable that disease germs are transferred from diseased to well persons by bedbugs and other insects that bite.

How yellow fever is transmitted

For a long time it was thought that yellow fever was carried through the air, but now it has been proved that yellow fever is not carried in this way. A well person can sleep with one who has yellow fever and not catch the disease. Yellow fever infection is carried from a yellow fever patient to a healthy person only by a certain mosquito. Keep this mosquito away from the yellow fever patients and there can be no spread of the disease.

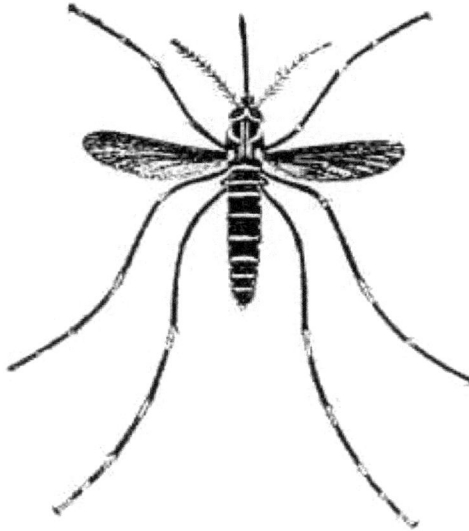

FIG. 48. The mosquito that carries yellow fever.

It is not many years since yellow fever was one of the most dreaded diseases in warm countries. To-day there is not the same fear of it, for the source of the disease has been discovered and practical methods have been devised to get rid of the mosquito which carries it.

How malaria is transmitted

Malarial fever is another disease transmitted by the bite of a mosquito, but the mosquito that carries malarial fever is not the same as the one that carries yellow fever. For a long time it was supposed that malaria came from the gases which rise from marshes. To-day it is known that it is not the gases that cause the sickness, but a mosquito which lives and grows in the marshes. Many countries that have heretofore been practically worthless on account of malarial fever, are being made valuable by draining the marshes and doing away with places where mosquitoes can hatch.

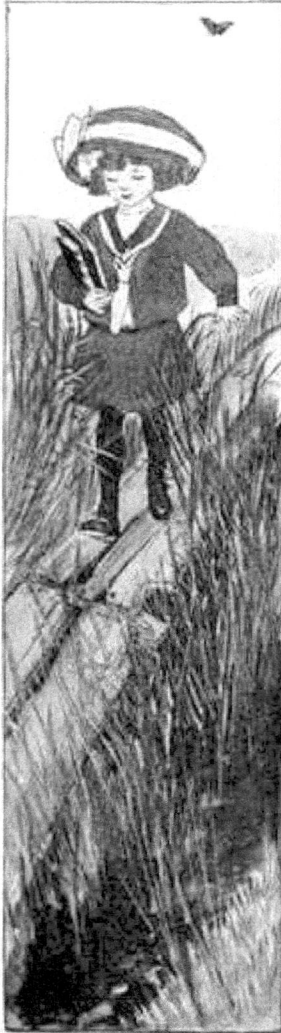

FIG. 49. One of the places where mosquitoes hatch.

How to get rid of the mosquito

It might seem a very hard task to get rid of mosquitoes in countries where there are so many of them; but it can be done. The mosquito must have still water in which to lay her eggs. In countries where there is danger of yellow fever or malaria, the rain barrel and the cistern should be screened, and the swamps and water holes filled up. Puddles of water should not be allowed to form anywhere, and low places where water might stand should be drained. By giving her no place in which to lay her eggs, we can get rid of the mosquito; and when the mosquito disappears, yellow fever and malaria disappear also.

How wood-ticks transmit disease

In certain portions of Montana, Washington, Idaho, Utah, and Wyoming, there is a peculiar disease known as Rocky Mountain spotted (tick) fever. It is now known that this disease is transmitted to people by the bite of a wood-tick. Not all wood-ticks carry this fever, and for people living in districts where this disease does not exist there is no danger in the bite of a wood-tick; but in a part of the country where the disease prevails, the wood-tick should be avoided.

How disease-bearing insects can be destroyed

All insects that are known to transmit diseases can be destroyed. If we will do away with stagnant water, the mosquito cannot hatch; if we will cut out underbrush and oil the domestic animals, the wood-tick will not find a place to grow. If we wish to get rid of disease, we must spend money and labor; but it is worth while, for human life is at stake.

Questions. 1. What insects are known to transmit diseases to man? 2. How is yellow fever transmitted? 3. Malarial fever? 4. What disease is transmitted by the wood-tick? 5. How can we get rid of the mosquito? 6. How can we get rid of ticks?

Remember. 1. It is a proved fact that diseases are transmitted to man by the bites of mosquitoes and wood-ticks. 2. It is possible to do away with both the mosquito and the wood-tick almost completely, although it requires a great deal of work and the expenditure of a large amount of money. 3. Health is the most valuable thing we have, and it is foolish to hesitate in giving the work and money necessary to exterminate disease-bearing insects, as well as the many other causes of sickness.

CHAPTER XXII

HOW TO KEEP GERMS OUT OF WOUNDS

How germs get through the skin

Germs get into our bodies through breaks in the skin. These breaks may be made by a cut or a scratch, by the bite of an insect, or even by the pulling out of a hair. There are some special germs, such as those which cause yellow fever, which are introduced by the bite of an insect; but at present we will consider only those germs that would naturally enter through any break in the skin.

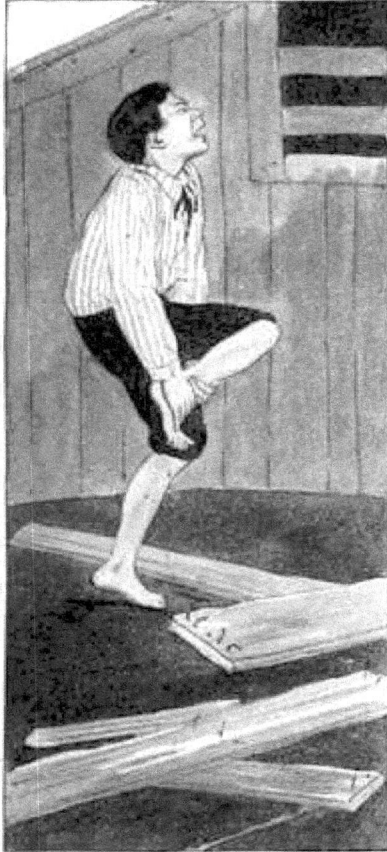

FIG. 50. Small, deep wounds are very liable to become infected.

The skin of the human body acts as an armor against certain germs that are constantly trying to get through it. There are several germs of this class. Some of them cause white pus, or matter, but this is the least dangerous kind of all. Another kind causes boils or even blood poisoning, and another kind causes erysipelas.

We cannot get rid of these germs, for they are everywhere, to a greater or less degree; but they are more abundant in dirty than in clean places. They cause every degree of inflammation, from a slight redness of the skin to the blood poisoning that brings death.

Real cause of suppuration

Sometimes you will hear people say that a wound suppurated (that is, became inflamed and full of matter) because the blood was in bad condition. As a matter of fact, there would have been no suppuration if germs had not got into the wound. It was not the condition of the blood that caused the suppuration, but the germs.

Sometimes, when only a few germs get into a wound, and when the cells of the body are all in good condition and doing their work properly, the suppuration will be very slight, because the healthy cells of the body will kill the germs. But if very many germs get in, even healthy body cells cannot kill them all.

We have said that the germs which cause suppuration are everywhere, so it would seem almost impossible to keep them out of a wound. This is true in a sense; but even after they have got into a wound, you can wash them out if you use plenty of soap and water to cleanse the wound thoroughly. When I said that it is impossible to keep them out of a wound, I meant an accidental wound, for it is quite possible to keep them out of a wound that is made intentionally, as is done by the surgeon.

How the surgeon prevents suppuration

Do you know how a surgeon gets ready to do an operation? The first thing he does is to see that the room is perfectly clean. He has the carpet taken up, the curtains taken down, and the floor and walls washed. This is to get rid of all the dirt and germs in the room. If you should look at the surgeon's instruments, so clean and bright, you would think it impossible for a germ to find a place to live on; but the surgeon knows how closely the germs cling, and therefore he boils all the instruments he is going to use. Then he puts the towels into a place where they are made so hot by steam that all the germs on them are killed. After everything in the room is perfectly clean, the surgeon cleans his patient with a very stiff brush, using plenty of soap and water which has been boiled to kill all the germs in it. He scrubs the part where the wound is to be made and the skin around it until it is red. Even then he is not satisfied, for he washes it off with alcohol and ether, to be sure that any germs that might be sticking in the fat are removed. He scrubs his hands in the same way. After all this is done, he can perform the operation without fear that any of the germs which cause suppuration will get in, for he knows that he has killed all of them that would touch the wound.

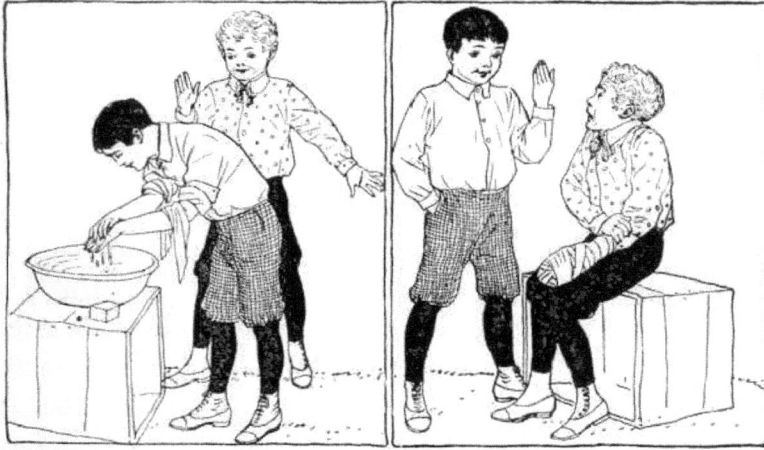

FIGS. 51 and 52. Always wash the simplest cut with soap and water; failure to do this may result in infection and much suffering.

How to prevent suppuration

Boys and girls cannot do all this before they cut their hands or skin their shins, but they can do the next best thing—they can keep their hands and the rest of their bodies clean at all times, and thus have as few germs on them as possible. Then, when they have cut themselves, they can go straight to some place where there is soap and water, and can wash the wound thoroughly. After this is done, a clean bandage should be placed on the cut part to prevent any other germs from getting in. If this is done every time you cut yourself, you will probably never have an infection—that is, a wound that suppurates.

Two boys were playing together one day. They ran into each other and each got a little cut on his hand. One boy went home at once, washed the wound, and put on a clean bandage. He lost a little time from his play, but was soon back and never had any trouble on account of the cut. The other boy thought it was foolish to quit his play to take care of such a little thing, so he tied his hand up in a dirty handkerchief. Two weeks later he was very ill. His arm was badly swollen and had to be cut open in several places; indeed, he came near losing his arm. It always pays to take care of a wound, be it never so slight.

Deep wounds made with small instruments, such as small knives, nails or toy pistols, are especially dangerous, because they are hard to clean and because they quickly heal up on the surface and leave the germs to grow at the bottom of the wound. Such wounds as these are dangerous for another reason.

Where germs of lockjaw grow

There is a germ that gets into wounds but does not cause suppuration. It is the germ of tetanus, or lockjaw. It lives in the ground, especially in the ground about barns, and its peculiar feature is that it will not grow in the air. If it gets into a large, open wound, it is easily killed, because it cannot grow where there is air. But when it gets into a small, deep wound where it cannot be reached, it stays there until the wound heals over on the surface, and then it begins to grow. It does not make the parts swell, as the germs of suppuration do, but quietly continues to grow, without the wound showing any sign of infection. Finally it develops a very severe poison that is taken up by the blood; then the victim suddenly begins to have spasms about the face, and finally these spasms extend to the entire body and kill him. Whenever you get a wound so deep that you cannot wash it thoroughly, go to a doctor and let him clean it out with some medicine that will kill the germs that cannot be reached by washing.

How boils are caused

Sometimes the germs that cause suppuration get under the skin at a point where a hair has been pulled out, or even work down beside the hair itself. When this happens, they cause suppuration under the skin, and the result is a boil. A boil is merely an infection with the germs that cause suppuration.

Questions. 1. How do germs get through the skin? 2. Can we get rid of all the germs that cause suppuration? 3. Why is it impossible for "bad blood" alone to cause suppuration? 4. How does the surgeon prevent suppuration? 5. How may you prevent suppuration? 6. What is the danger of cutting corns with an ordinary knife or razor? 7. Where do germs of lockjaw grow? 8. What causes boils?

Remember. 1. Germs and not "bad blood" are the cause of suppuration. 2. Always keep as clean as possible, and immediately wash any cut, no matter how small. 3. If you have a deep wound, go at once to a doctor, and let him clean it out and kill the germs that may be at the bottom of the wound.

CHAPTER XXIII

TRANSMISSION OF DIPHTHERIA

How germs may cause sickness without entering the body

Some germs that cause disease do not get into the body, but grow upon its surface, that is, they grow on the mucous membranes—the skin of the mouth, the throat, and the nose. As they grow, they develop poisons that are absorbed by the body, and that make us very sick. The germs that cause diphtheria belong to this class.

Prevalence of diphtheria

Diphtheria is one of the most common of all the preventable diseases. It causes more deaths than any of the other diseases that can be prevented, except tuberculosis. The great prevalence of diphtheria is due to lack of care on the part of those who have this disease and of those who come in contact with them.

Where the diphtheria germ comes from

The germ that causes diphtheria always comes from some person or animal that has diphtheria. It never "just happens." If you went into your yard in the morning and found some beets growing in your flower bed, you would know positively that beet seeds had got into your flower bed in some way. You would not say that the beets just happened to grow there. So diphtheria will not "just happen." Diphtheria is always caused by germs that come from some one who has diphtheria. They may have come in a letter that was written in the room with the sick person. They may have come from the library in a book that had been used by some one ill with diphtheria. They may have come on some toy that had been played with by a child that had the disease. There are a thousand ways by which the germs may be brought to you without your knowing where they come from.

How to confine diphtheria germs

The public health officers try hard to keep these germs from being brought to you. In order to do this, they have to shut away from other people those who have diphtheria germs; that is, they make the sick ones stay at home until they are free from the germs of the disease. We call this *quarantine.* Quarantine means that you must stay away from other people when you are sick with a communicable disease, and that other people must stay away from you. People are not put in quarantine because they are sick, but because they are dangerous, and because we are trying to prevent other people from getting the same disease. Do not think the health officers unreasonable when they tell you that you must stay at home and that no one can come in to see you. This is done to protect other people and to keep them from getting the same disease that you have. If you ever have diphtheria, or any other communicable disease, you must remember that if any of your playmates come in to see you, they may get the same disease.

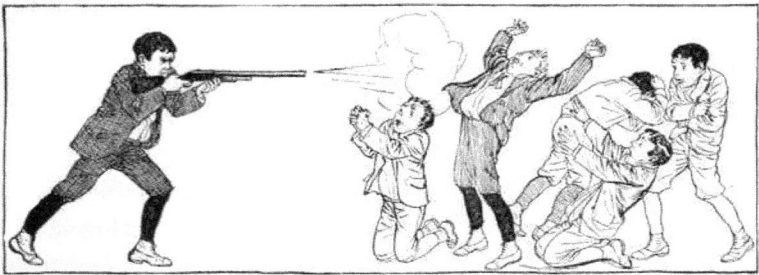

FIG. 53. Disease germs are as deadly as guns.

Seriousness of breaking quarantine

Diphtheria kills a great many children, and to play with your friends after you have had diphtheria, and before the health officer tells you that you may, is almost like trying to kill them. They might be very sick and die, or they might be very sick and get well, or they might not be sick at all; but you never can tell what will happen if they are exposed to the disease. If you were to take a gun and shoot at a friend, you might kill him, or you might shoot his leg off, or you might not hit him at all; but you would be trying to hit him, and it would not be your fault if you did not. It is just the same if you play with a friend when you have a communicable disease; you shoot the disease germ at him, and if you do not hit him, it is not your fault.

Why quarantine is not raised sooner

Sometimes people who have been sick with a communicable disease feel perfectly well, but the health officer tells them he cannot let them out of quarantine. This is because he knows that such people still have in their bodies the germs that cause the disease, and that as long as these germs are there they can give the disease to other people. It is not pleasant to have to stay in quarantine when you feel that you are well, and children, as well as older people, are very likely to become restless under the circumstances. You see an illustration of such a patient in Figure 60, where the little girl, who is under quarantine for scarlet fever, but who is feeling quite well, is giving a book to two of her friends. The book contains the germs that cause scarlet fever, and the boys are very likely to contract the disease by handling the book.

Why some cases of diphtheria escape quarantine:

(1) From failure to detect mild cases

If every case of diphtheria were quarantined, and the people obeyed the health officer, there would soon be no more diphtheria. But how does it happen that every case of diphtheria is not quarantined? Diphtheria is a very peculiar disease. Sometimes it makes people so sick that they die in spite of everything that can be done for them; sometimes it makes the throat only a little sore, and the child seems so slightly ill that his mother says to herself, "He is fretful," and does not call the doctor. In the latter case the child often keeps on going to school, and exposes other children to the disease; some of them catch it, and become very sick or even die. In still other cases, the mother thinks that a child has only a case of tonsillitis and does not call a doctor; the child's brothers and sisters go to school and may carry the germs to other children. I have known a great many cases of diphtheria to be spread in this way.

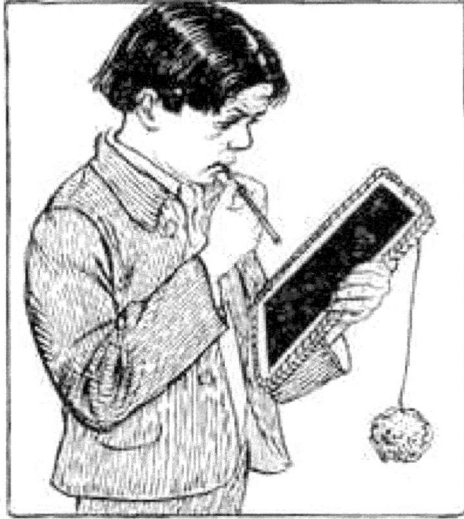

FIG. 54. The old, insanitary slates and sponges have gone out of use, but many people of to-day still follow the dangerous habit of putting pencils into their mouths.

Sometimes a dairyman thinks that his child has nothing more serious than tonsillitis, and goes on selling milk. A great many epidemics have resulted from such cases. Sore throats should not be treated lightly, for the most severe forms of diphtheria may develop from germs that come from a throat that is only slightly sore. If there is a case of diphtheria in the town where you live, and if your throat feels the least bit sore, have your doctor examine it at once. If you do not wish to have your family doctor look at your throat, go to the health officer. Had you not rather stay at home for a week or two than see your best friends ill or dead because of your carelessness?

(2) From diphtheria germs in throats that are not sore

There is another peculiar thing about the germ of diphtheria. It will often get into a throat and grow a little, just enough to keep alive, but without making the throat sore at all. The person in whose throat the germs are will have no idea that they are there, but when he comes in contact with some one who has a delicate throat, he may give diphtheria to that person. The disease does not develop in some throats because the body cells are all healthy and doing their work so well that, when the diphtheria germs try to take hold, they are driven off and not allowed to grow. This is the reason that, before he raises the quarantine, the careful health officer takes a "culture" from the throat of everyone in a house where there has been diphtheria.

How mild cases may be detected

The health officer takes a culture by wiping the throat with a little cotton on a long stick, which he then puts down into a long glass tube containing some substance that diphtheria germs like to grow on. If there are any diphtheria germs in the throat, they will soon show on this culture material. Then the health officer will say, "No, we cannot let you out yet, for the germs are still in your throat." No person who has been staying in a house where there is diphtheria should be allowed to go out until a culture proves that his throat is free from the germs of diphtheria.

You see how hard it is to quarantine all cases of diphtheria, when children are sometimes allowed even to go to school with sore throats that are really diphtheritic. Only two things are necessary for getting rid of diphtheria: one is to quarantine every case, and the other, to have the people do just what they are told when under quarantine. This latter is just as important as the quarantine itself, for people often do not obey the health officer's directions. Now let us see what are some of these directions.

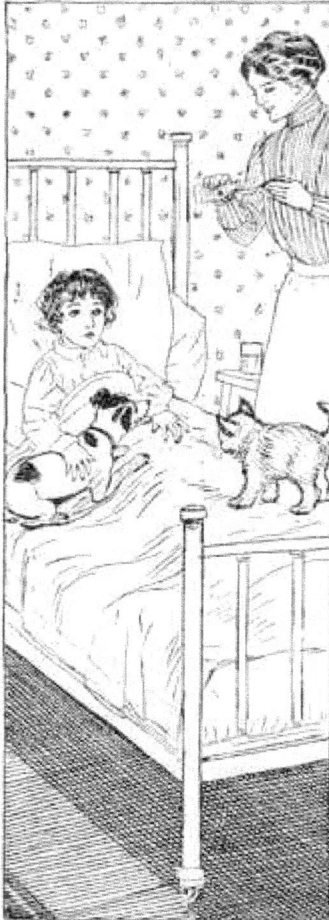

FIG. 55. How pets may become carriers of disease.

If you are the patient, the health officer will say that you must be put in a room where there is just enough furniture to make you comfortable, and that no one except the nurse and the doctor is to go into that room. He will say that the nurse must stay in your room all the time, or that she must at least not go into any other room in the house; that your meals must be left outside your door, and that the person who brings them must go away before the door is opened by the nurse. Furthermore, as everything in the room that cannot be boiled, or otherwise disinfected, will have to be burned when you are well, your pet books and toys had better not be taken in.

Finally, nothing is to be carried from the room until it has been put into a solution that will kill the germs, and this means not only dishes, bedding, and clothing, but even books and letters. The nurse must see that all discharges from the throat and nose are received on little cloths, which are to be burned immediately.

How quarantine rules are broken

These are the things that the health officer will tell your parents must be done. Now let us see what sometimes happens. Your mother will want to see her little child so much that she cannot wait until you are well, so she will slip into your room, kiss your forehead, and hold you tight against her. When a little later she kisses your baby brother, and is so thankful that he is not sick too, she does not realize that she is kissing the very same disease into his little throat. Or, perhaps your mother is the nurse, and in the night she hears your little brother crying; she thinks, "Surely I can slip out and just cover him up; it will not hurt him just for once," and she does so. What happens? In a few days your doctor tells you that your little brother will have to come in and stay with you.

Perhaps your father grows anxious to see you, and one morning he says he cannot stand it another minute, so he slips in for a few moments before going to business. In a few days one of his clerks fails to come to work. Your father sends a messenger to see what the trouble is, and the word comes back, "He has diphtheria." Then your father says, "What are these health officers doing that they do not stop this thing?" He is very indignant, but it never occurs to him that he himself has spread the disease by doing just what he promised the health officer he would not do.

How dogs and cats carry disease germs

The doctor told your mother not to take anything from the room until it had been disinfected. But you do not consider Towser, your dog, and Tabby, your cat, "anything," so you persuade your mother to let them come in, and you have a good play with them. You let them rub against your face and romp on your bed, and do everything that pet dogs and cats like to do, and in the meantime their fur is getting full of diphtheria germs. Then Towser and Tabby run out-of-doors and play with the boys and girls of the neighborhood. Soon the parents are wondering why the health officers do not stop the spread of the disease. No dog or cat should ever be permitted to come into a house where there is a contagious disease.

These are not all the ways in which people disobey the orders of the health officer and of the doctor, but these are enough to show you that it is a very important thing to do just what they tell you. It is not always easy to follow all these rules, but it is far better to follow these, and many more, than to have to think that you have caused the death of either a friend or a stranger.

Questions. 1. How does the poison of diphtheria get into the system? 2. Where does the diphtheria germ come from? 3. What is quarantine? 4. What is the danger in breaking quarantine? 5. Why is quarantine continued after you feel well? 6. How does it happen that some cases of diphtheria are not quarantined? 7. What is a diphtheria culture? 8. What rules should you observe while in quarantine? 9. Tell some of the ways by which quarantine is broken. 10. How do pet dogs and cats sometimes get disease germs?

Remember. 1. The germs that cause diphtheria always come from some person or animal that carries diphtheria germs. 2. Diphtheria is always caused by the diphtheria germ, and the diphtheria germ cannot cause any other disease. 3. People are quarantined to prevent other people from getting the disease. 4. If there is diphtheria in your neighborhood, and your throat becomes sore, have the doctor examine it. 5. Every person who has been staying in a house where there is a case of diphtheria should have his throat examined to make sure he is not carrying germs. 6. Never play with dogs or cats when you have a contagious disease. 7. People who do not obey quarantine regulations cause a great deal of suffering and many deaths.

CHAPTER XXIV

THE CURE OF DIPHTHERIA

Nature of diphtheria poison

The germs of diphtheria do not get into the blood through the skin, but grow on the surface of the mucous membrane (skin of the throat), and there produce a poison that gets into the blood through this membrane. It is this poison that makes you sick, and it is called a *toxin*. You already know that when people have diphtheria, they are sometimes very sick and sometimes only slightly sick, and that the germ can live in some throats without causing any ill effects whatever.

How diphtheria toxin is fought

As soon as the diphtheria germ begins to grow in a throat, the little cells of the body begin to make a certain substance and to pour it into the blood. This substance we call *antitoxin*, which means opposed to the toxin in the blood. If the little cells make the substance fast enough, the germs will stop growing, or in some cases they never really get started growing, because they cannot exist where there is much antitoxin. Antitoxin looks like clear water. The following experiment will show you something that acts in very much the same way that antitoxin does.

If you take a solution of litmus that is made alkaline, it will be very blue, like indigo; but if you drop a few drops of lemon juice into this solution it will turn red. Lemon juice is acid, and is just the opposite of alkali. Now, if you put a few drops of ammonia, which is alkali, into the red solution, it will turn blue again. If you put a little more lemon juice, very carefully, drop by drop, into the blue solution, it will gradually turn lighter, until it is entirely clear.

How antitoxin acts

We will suppose that the blue is due to the toxin produced by the diphtheria germ, and that the lemon juice is the antitoxin produced by the cells in the body. If the antitoxin is made fast enough, the blue disappears; but if the toxin is made faster than the antitoxin, the blue remains. It is the same way in the body, only it is not litmus and acids and alkalies that we have to deal with. If the toxin is made faster than the antitoxin, the germs grow, and we get sicker and sicker; but if the antitoxin is made faster than the toxin, then the germs cannot grow, and we soon get well, or perhaps do not get sick at all.

How antitoxin was discovered

Doctors knew that this was what happened, but for a great many years they could not discover the composition of the antitoxin that is made in the body. One day a doctor suggested, "If we cannot find out the chemical nature of this thing that is made in the body, why can we not make it in the body of some animal and then use the blood of the animal?" And that is just what they did. They put diphtheria germs into beef tea, and let them grow very fast and make all the toxin they could. Then the doctors strained the germs out by passing the beef tea through a fine filter, in this way getting the poison, and not the germs. Then they gave a strong, healthy horse a small quantity of this poison; they did not feed it to him, but injected it into his blood. Of course the horse was sick for a while, but soon he began to get well again, for the cells in his body immediately went to work making antitoxin.

When the horse was well, the doctors gave him more of the poison; this time he was not so sick and got well even more quickly. This treatment with toxin was repeated in gradually increasing doses until the poison did not affect the horse at all. Then the doctors said, "His blood is full of antitoxin, and we will see what it will do when injected into some other animal." So they drew off some of the horse's blood and took out all the little red cells, leaving nothing but the clear fluid of the blood. They planted diphtheria germs in a rabbit's throat, and when the rabbit became very sick, they gave him some of the antitoxin from the horse. The rabbit immediately got well. Afterward they gave some of this antitoxin to a little boy who was very sick with diphtheria, and he, too, got well. Ever since then the doctors have been saving many lives by the use of antitoxin.

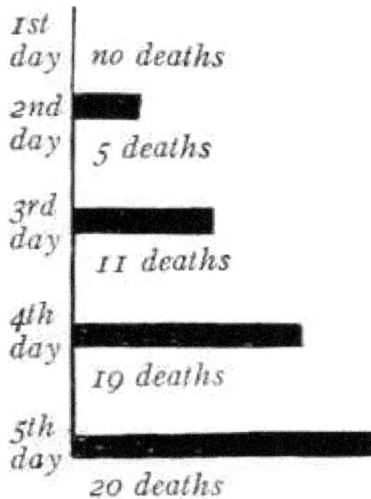

FIG. 56. Showing the number of deaths in 100 cases of diphtheria when antitoxin is used on the first, second, third, fourth, and fifth days.

Evidences that antitoxin saves lives

Someone may ask, "How do we know that it is the antitoxin that saves lives?" In just this way: before we knew anything about antitoxin, about half of all the people with diphtheria died; but since we have had antitoxin, only about twelve die out of every hundred who have this disease. More than this, we know that when the antitoxin is given within the first twenty-four hours after the patient is taken sick, there is only about one death for every one thousand cases of diphtheria. Do you not think that this is strong proof that antitoxin saves lives?

How antitoxin saves lives

Antitoxin saves lives not only by curing those who have diphtheria, but by preventing others from having it. If a person who has been where there is a case of diphtheria is given a dose of antitoxin, he will not have the disease, because his blood will contain enough antitoxin to destroy the diphtheria toxin present. If you will watch a careful doctor when he makes his first visit to a case of diphtheria, you will notice that, as soon as he gets through treating the patient, he gives all members of the family who have been near the patient a dose of antitoxin to keep them from getting sick.

Antitoxin not a poison

Some people may tell you that antitoxin is a poison and should not be used. The statement that it is in itself a poison is true. But it is also true that in your body there are many things that would poison you if you got too much of them. For instance, there is a gland in your throat (the thyroid) which secretes a substance that is necessary for your health, but if you were to take the secretion of ten such glands it would kill you at once. Now, if the cells in your body make antitoxin when you have diphtheria, it is probable that antitoxin is the very thing needed. And if you can help these cells by giving them antitoxin, ready-made, does it not seem a reasonable thing to do? People who give the name of poison to a substance which is known to have saved many lives are not worthy of attention. Anything may prove a poison if taken in excess; too much play will prove a poison, and too much work also.

Questions. 1. What is the poison of diphtheria called? 2. What is antitoxin? 3. Compare the action of antitoxin on the blood with the action of an acid on the litmus solution. 4. Tell about the discovery of antitoxin. 5. How do we know that antitoxin saves lives? 6. How does antitoxin prevent diphtheria? 7. Why should antitoxin not be regarded as a poison?

Remember. 1. Antitoxin is what the cells in your body make when you have diphtheria. 2. By using the antitoxin taken from a horse, you save your own cells the struggle necessary to make it fast enough to kill the diphtheria germs. 3. If you have diphtheria, and antitoxin is given promptly, you will get well. 4. If you have been exposed to diphtheria, antitoxin will prevent your having the disease. 5. Antitoxin is no more a poison than are many other medicines.

CHAPTER XXV

HOW TYPHOID FEVER GERMS ARE CARRIED

How typhoid fever germs get into the system

There are certain diseases, the germs of which get into bodies through our mouths. That is, we eat or drink them. Some of these diseases are typhoid fever, cholera, the summer complaints of children, tuberculosis, and diphtheria. At present we shall learn about the germ that causes typhoid fever, how it gets into our food and drink, and how we may prevent the disease by getting rid of this germ.

Typhoid fever, like all other diseases caused by germs, is caused by one kind of germ, and one kind only. You cannot get typhoid fever by eating cholera germs any more than you can get diphtheria from typhoid germs.

Animals free from typhoid

So far as we know, there is no animal except man that has typhoid fever. Since the germs of any disease must come from an animal suffering from that disease, and as man is the only animal that has typhoid fever, it naturally follows that the only way to get typhoid fever is from some person who has the fever or has had it.

How typhoid germs leave the body

We know that typhoid fever germs get into the body with food, but how do they get out? Once in a great while germs are found in the matter that the patient vomits, or spits up, but this is a rare occurrence, so rare that we need hardly consider it. The germs are present in the blood of the sufferer, but other people do not get his blood on their hands or in their food. There are two things that come from the patient that are loaded with these germs, and these are the urine and bowel discharges. In these two excretions of the body are found practically all the typhoid germs that come from the patient, and these are the causes of other infections. In other words, it is from these two excretions that the germs get into food and drink.

How do the typhoid germs get into our food? What is done with the excretions after they come from the body? You will probably say that the nurse throws them into the sewer. Very true; but where do they go when they are thrown into the sewer? The sewer must empty somewhere, and in most instances it empties into a stream, the water of which is used for drinking purposes.

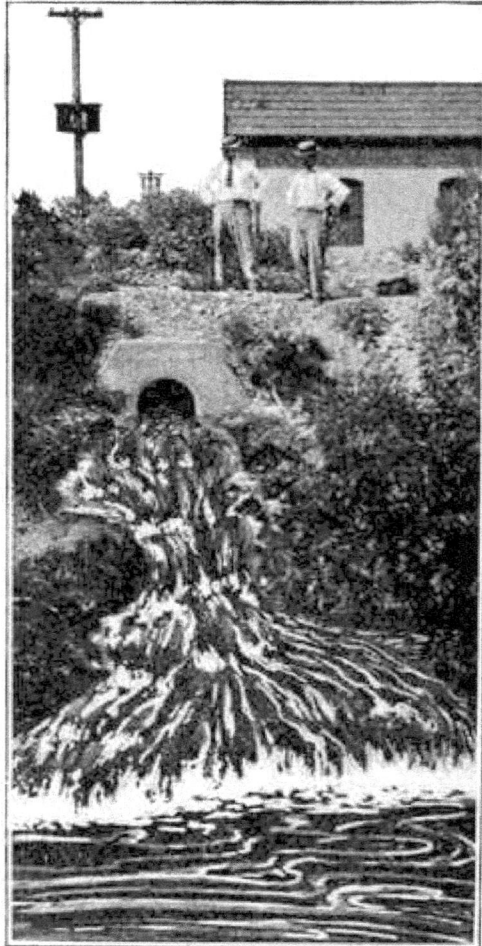

FIG. 57. Pollution of a stream with sewage.

The widespread evil due to the sickness of one person

You may think that the germs from one person would not make much difference, but that is where you are mistaken. There is a town in Pennsylvania of about eight thousand inhabitants, which gets its water from a stream that flows down from the mountains. One cold winter, while the stream was frozen, a man living on the bank of the stream was taken sick with typhoid fever. His nurse threw the urine and the discharges from his bowels on the ice on the bank of the creek. When the ice melted, the typhoid germs in the discharges found their way to the stream that furnished drinking water to people farther down, and in a very short time there were over one thousand cases of typhoid fever in that town. Before the ice melted there had not been a single case of typhoid, and every one of the thousand cases came from the water into which had been allowed to flow the discharges from one man with typhoid fever. You see what germs from one person may do.

How long typhoid fever germs live in a stream

Sometimes people say that a stream purifies itself every few miles. It does purify itself of some things, but disease germs live from twenty-five to thirty-five days in water, and a stream flows a long way in thirty days.

The pollution of streams with sewage

Sometimes we hear people say that it is safe to put sewage into a certain stream, because no town uses that stream for drinking water. But of this they can never be sure. Not long ago certain people said that the water from the river which flowed through their town was used only by two dairymen and a vegetable gardener, and therefore there was no danger in running sewage into the stream. Yet the dairymen and the gardener sold all their produce in that very town. The townspeople never considered that the water into which they ran their sewage was used by the dairymen for washing their milk vessels (and perhaps for diluting the milk), and by the gardener for washing his lettuce and other vegetables. Thus the germs of disease were brought directly back to the town.

Do not think that you are safe in polluting a stream with sewage because no town uses the water from that stream. The individual on the farm is entitled to protection just as much as the individual in the town. Always remember that when you pollute with disease the water used by the farmer, he may bring that disease back into the town with the produce of his farm.

No sewage, no matter how small the amount, should ever be permitted to go into a stream until all the disease germs it contains have been killed. This can be done, though it will cost something; but we cannot get rid of disease germs without work, and work cannot be done without being paid for.

There are other ways of scattering typhoid germs besides running sewage into streams. Sometimes the nurse does not throw the discharges from a typhoid fever patient into a sewer at all, but into a closet vault. Remember how the material from a closet vault goes through open ground into a well, and you will understand what happens. The germs get into the well, and the whole family may then have typhoid fever.

Let us suppose that the nurse did not throw the discharges either into the closet or into the sewer, but carelessly threw them out on the ground behind the house, where, as it was winter time, they froze as hard as rocks. It does not seem to hurt typhoid germs in the least to be frozen; when they get warm again they are as lively as ever. Let us suppose these particular germs lay there all winter, but in the spring when everything melted the germs were still alive and ready to spread disease. It happened that they did not get into the well or into the milk, but they did get on your food, and made you ill with typhoid fever.

How flies carry typhoid germs

How did the germs get to your food? About the time that the germs were thawed out, and were beginning to double in number every hour or two, along came a fly and thought that spot an attractive one for a lunch. Accordingly he walked over this mass of filth, collecting a supply of germs on his feet, and then came in and tracked them over your bread and butter or other food.

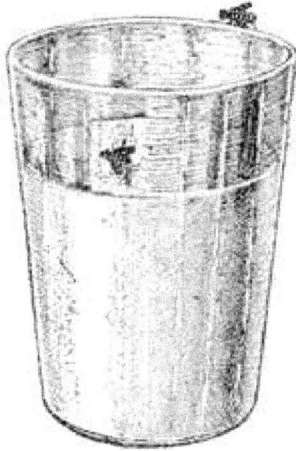

FIG. 58. Flies crawling on the edge of the glass or falling into the milk leave germs that cause disease.

How typhoid germs get into milk

That is how you got the fever; but the trouble did not stop with you. When you fell sick, your father thought it was time to clean the yard, but he was not very careful what he did with the dirt, including the typhoid fever discharges which the nurse threw out on the snow during the winter. There was a low place in the barnyard and there he dumped the dirt. One of the cows thought this fresh pile of dirt would make a comfortable place to lie down in. The next morning the milkman milked her without first washing her sides and udder, and hundreds of little particles of dirt, each one loaded with germs, fell into the milk. The milk from all the cows was mixed together, and by the time it got to town these germs had grown into many thousands. Some of the people who drank the milk became ill with typhoid fever and wondered afterward where they had taken this disease.

Why the recovered patient is dangerous

The discharges from a typhoid fever patient contain typhoid germs not only while the disease lasts, but for many months after the patient is well. In some cases they are present for years after the illness is over.

The story of the careless nurses

Here is a story about typhoid fever that illustrates the importance of washing and boiling everything that comes from a sickroom. A few years ago there was an epidemic of typhoid fever in a certain town. One of the hospitals was very much crowded, and it became necessary to employ several extra nurses. All the nurses knew the importance of washing their hands after handling the patients, and the old nurses had seen so many bad results from failure to observe this rule that they were very careful. Three of the new nurses, however, thought it a great deal of trouble to be washing their hands all the time, so more and more they neglected this important duty. The result was that all three of these girls got typhoid fever and died. They paid the penalty for neglecting the duty that they well knew they should have performed.

Typhoid fever can be wiped out by attention to neglected details—that is, by disinfecting discharges before throwing them away; by disposing of excretions only in places that are made for them; by adding lime to the closet vault every day to kill any germs present; by making the closet in such a way that flies cannot get into it; and by not permitting sewage to enter any stream until all the disease germs have been killed. All these things can be done. It will require a little work; but had you not rather take a little extra care than run the risk of catching or spreading typhoid fever?

Questions. 1. How do typhoid fever germs get into the body? 2. What is one source of these germs? 3. How do these germs leave the body? 4. Name several ways by which typhoid germs in a stream may get into foods. 5. How do flies carry typhoid fever germs? 6. How do these germs get into milk?

Remember. 1. Typhoid germs come from people who have typhoid fever; they are found in the urine and bowel discharges. 2. No one should ever answer Nature's calls except in a place provided for that purpose. 3. No sewage should be allowed to go into any stream until all the germs in it have been killed. 4. Disease germs will live in running water fully as long as they will in still water. 5. The discharges from a single person may infect a whole city. 6. When typhoid fever germs get into milk, they grow very rapidly; hundreds of people have been given typhoid fever by drinking the milk from a dairy where there was a single person sick with this disease. 7. People who have had typhoid often carry the germs for several months after they are well.

CHAPTER XXVI

HOOKWORM DISEASE AND AMOEBIC DYSENTERY

Hookworm disease and amoebic dysentery resemble typhoid fever in one respect, in that they, too are spread by the improper disposal of human excreta.

Where hookworm disease prevails

Hookworm disease is found almost exclusively in tropical or subtropical climates. In the United States it is rarely seen north of the Potomac and Ohio rivers.

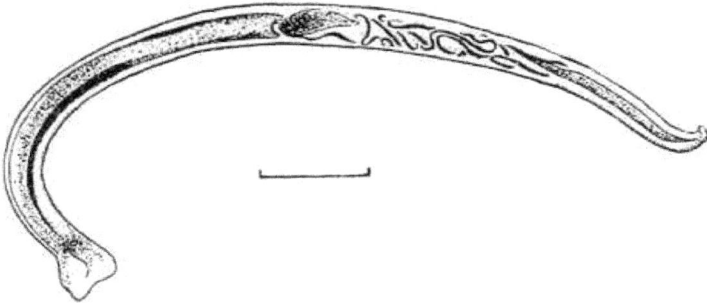

FIG. 59. A full-grown hookworm, magnified; the short line shows the average length of the hookworm.

What the hookworm is

This disease is not caused by a germ, as is typhoid fever, but by a worm from a quarter to half an inch long, and about as thick as a small hairpin. These worms get into a person's intestinal canal, and there lay their eggs, which are later given off in the bowel discharges. When these discharges are thrown on the ground, or are put into an open water-closet, they may be carried about by chickens, flies, and pigs. Then the eggs hatch in the soil and tiny hookworms result. When human excreta are not properly disposed of, in climates where hookworm disease prevails, the soil becomes practically full of these little worms, and from the soil they find their way into the bodies of the people.

How it enters the body

There are two principal ways by which the hookworm may enter the body. One is through the mouth, which these worms reach in practically the same way as do typhoid fever germs. The hookworm may enter the body through the skin also. Some authorities state that the worm bores its way in; but it is probable that it does not actually bore through sound skin, but enters at some point where there is a small break.

Where it lives in the body

After the worm gets through the skin, it is taken into the blood and carried to the lungs, and from there it finds its way to the throat and is swallowed. It makes no difference whether the hookworm is swallowed or enters the body through the skin; it finally reaches the intestinal canal, where it then makes its home. Sometimes thousands of these worms are found in a single person, and each one of them entered the body through the mouth or through the skin. The worms do not multiply in the body, and the eggs they lay never hatch until after they have left the body.

How it affects the patient

When the hookworm gets into the intestinal canal, it fastens itself to the wall and sucks the blood from it, at the same time giving off a poison that enters the blood of the victim. The loss of blood and the effects of the poison soon cause the person in whose body these worms are living to become weak, pale, and thin. He is not able to do much work, if any, and the result is that people suffering from this disease are often called lazy. They are not lazy; they are sick, and many of them die.

How hookworm disease can be prevented

All this sickness and all these deaths might be prevented simply by the proper disposal of human excreta. No human excreta should ever be put anywhere except into a properly constructed sewer or properly constructed privy. If this rule were always observed, both hookworm disease and typhoid fever would be abolished.

Where amoebic dysentery prevails

Amoebic dysentery is another disease that is confined almost entirely to tropical and subtropical climates, though cases sometimes occur in colder regions.

How it is spread and how it may be prevented

This disease, like typhoid fever, is caused by a germ that leaves the body with the bowel discharges. The germ makes its way into the body in the same way that the typhoid germ enters; that is, it is taken in with food or drink. The various means by which this germ gets into our food are the same as those by which the typhoid germ gets in; and the precautions that will prevent the spread of typhoid fever will also prevent dysentery. Amoebic dysentery kills a great many people in warm climates, though it does not kill as many as does typhoid fever. If it does not cause immediate death, it often leaves the patient very weak and sickly for months or years.

Questions. 1. In what climates are hookworm disease and amoebic dysentery commonly found? 2. In what respects do they resemble typhoid fever? 3. How does the hookworm enter the body? 4. Where do the hookworm eggs hatch? 5. How can hookworm disease be prevented? 6. What other diseases can be prevented by the same precautions?

Remember. 1. Typhoid fever, hookworm disease, and amoebic dysentery are all caused by the improper disposal of human excreta. 2. Most of the sickness that can be prevented is the result of dirty habits; if all people would keep clean and see that everything about them was kept clean, a great deal of sickness would be prevented and a great many lives would be saved.

CHAPTER XXVII

HOW SCARLET FEVER IS CARRIED

There are certain diseases that we know to be communicable (that is, "catching"), but as yet we do not know the germ that causes them, and therefore we cannot tell just how they are carried about. We do know that they are transferred from one person to another; but not being able to locate the cause, as we can in the diseases of which we do know the germ, we cannot explain how it is done.

How scarlet fever is like diphtheria

Among the diseases of this class we find scarlet fever. In one respect scarlet fever acts much the same as diphtheria. A person may have it and not be very sick, sometimes hardly sick at all. At night a child may have a high fever, with a slightly sore throat, and the next morning he may feel perfectly well. The mother supposes that the fever was due to an "upset stomach," thinks no more about it, and sends the child to school. The next time the child takes a bath, he perhaps notices that the skin peels off over some parts of the body. This means that the high fever was due to scarlet fever, but the breaking-out (rash) was so fine that it was not noticed. It also means that all the children in the school have been exposed to the disease. These very mild cases are the most dangerous because so often they are not recognized.

Why mild cases are dangerous:

(1) For the severe cases they cause

There are two things to be remembered in connection with these mild forms of scarlet fever, as well as of every other communicable disease. The first is that the same cause which produces a mild form of the disease in one child may produce its most severe form in another child. You can contract a mild form of the disease from exposure to a severe case; and you can contract a severe form from exposure to a mild case. The character of the case to which you are exposed will give no indication of the form the disease will assume in your body.

(2) For the bad after effects

The next thing to be remembered about the mild form of scarlet fever is that, though the child may not be made very sick at the time, there may later be very bad results. A child who has had scarlet fever in such a mild form that he hardly knew he was sick, may, for a while, appear to be quite well; then suddenly he has an earache, and an abscess forms. This abscess is due to the scarlet fever germs which have gone from the throat to the ear, and as a result the child may lose his hearing entirely.

The child may not, perhaps, have an abscess, but after a time he may begin to lose flesh, and to grow pale. He does not care for his meals, does not care to play, says he is tired, and wants to lie still all the time. Finally his mother thinks it might be a good idea to have a doctor see him. The doctor examines his body carefully, and then asks for a sample of his urine. When he has examined this, he looks very serious and asks the mother when the child was sick last, and what the disease was. Perhaps she has forgotten all about the slight attack of fever, and the doctor must question her very carefully before she recalls it. At length it occurs to her, and then the doctor asks, "After this attack of fever, did you notice that the skin came off his hands and body?" She replies that she did, and then the doctor tells her that the child really had scarlet fever, and, owing to lack of care, he now has kidney disease. This is a very serious trouble, from which he may never recover, or, in case of recovery, he may always be weak and sickly. Even a mild attack of scarlet fever is not to be neglected; it is a severe and dangerous disease in its very mildest form. It not only kills a great many boys and girls, but it makes delicate in health for all their lives many of those who apparently recover.

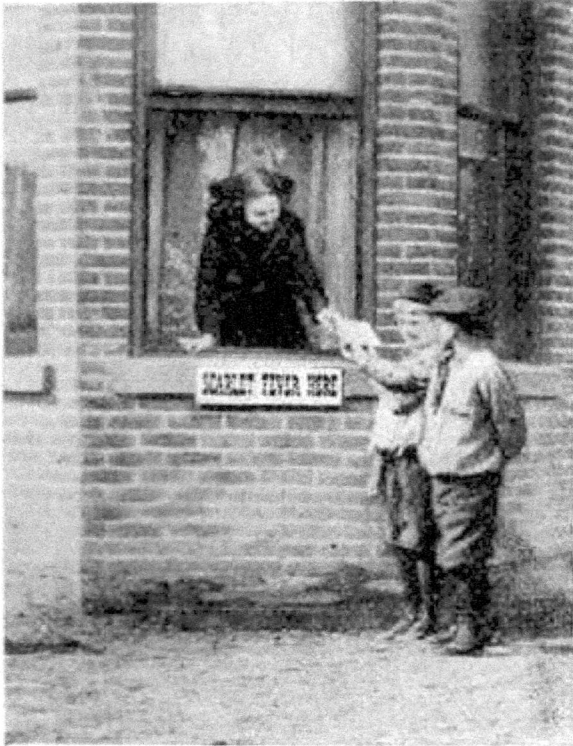

FIG. 60. One of the ways by which quarantine is broken.

How confusion of names causes mild cases to go undetected

We often hear people speak of two diseases which they think are not scarlet fever. These two diseases are scarlatina and scarlet rash. Now scarlatina is simply the scientific name for scarlet fever. Some doctors will tell you that you have scarlatina and that it is not exactly scarlet fever. A doctor who says this either is deceiving you or does not know any better. In either case, he ought not to be a doctor, for he lets children be exposed to a disease that is likely to kill many of them. It is the same with scarlet rash. This, too, is simply another name for scarlet fever. Changing the name does not change the disease, and you may call it scarlet fever, scarlatina, or scarlet rash—it makes no difference which; the disease is one and the same.

Why quarantine is necessary for scarlet fever

Quarantine is the only way known for preventing the spread of scarlet fever, as well as of diphtheria. If every case of scarlet fever were quarantined, we could soon stop this disease; but every case is not quarantined, because some of them are so mild that they are not recognized.

How breaking quarantine shows selfishness

Even when a case is quarantined, the people sometimes neglect the instructions given, just as they do when there is a case of diphtheria. Then there are cases that are known to be scarlet fever but are not reported to the health officers, because the people do not want to be quarantined. They simply do not want to be put to any inconvenience themselves, and although this seems a very strange way for people to act, it happens very often. There are many selfish people in the world; there are even people who will not report a case of scarlet fever because to do so might prevent their going to a party. Selfishness is at the bottom of it.

It is extremely important that a child should be absolutely free from all the little scales of skin which are thrown off after scarlet fever, before he returns to school or mingles again with others. If there is a discharge from the nose or ears after the scales have disappeared from the skin, there is still danger of spreading the disease, for these discharges often retain the infection for many months.

Questions. 1. Give two reasons why mild cases of scarlet fever should be carefully treated. 2. Why is quarantine necessary? 3. How does selfishness lead people to spread scarlet fever? 4. When is it safe to let a scarlet fever patient mingle with well people?

Remember. 1. If you have scarlet fever and are not very sick, do not think that you will not be dangerous to others; severe cases sometimes come from exposure to the mildest cases. 2. Mild cases of scarlet fever often leave very bad results, if the patient is not cared for. 3. Be very careful until you are entirely well. 4. Scarlatina and scarlet rash are nothing but scarlet fever; keep away from people who have them. 5. Quarantine is the only way by which we can prevent the spread of scarlet fever; there is no medicine that will prevent it. 6. People who violate quarantine regulations are both selfish and stupid.

CHAPTER XXVIII

MEASLES AND WHOOPING COUGH DANGEROUS DISEASES

Measles is a disease in the same class as scarlet fever. We do not know the cause, but we do know that it is communicable.

Why measles should be avoided

Measles is usually not a severe disease; that is, it does not kill as many persons in proportion to the number of cases as does scarlet fever. It does, however, kill more people than most of us think; a great many little babies die of it. How often we hear mothers say, "I wish my children would have measles and be done with it." It would be very convenient if they could have measles in a mild way and "be done with it." The trouble is, that we cannot tell whether it will take a mild form, and, worse than this, we do not know when they will be done with it.

If you should go into the children's wards of a large hospital, you would know why measles should be avoided. There you would hear the doctors questioning the mothers about the previous diseases of the little ones. You would be surprised at the number who replied, "He has not had anything but measles." Then you would hear the question, "How long since he had the measles?" "He was just over it when he was taken sick with this trouble." What is "this trouble"? Follow the doctor along from bed to bed and see the cases of pneumonia that started when the child "was just over measles"; see how many cases of empyema (abscess in the chest) began just after the measles ended; how many cases of abscess in the bone, how many cases of disease of the kidneys appeared after the child recovered from the measles. Then go down into the eye and ear wards and see how many diseased eyes and ears have followed an attack of the measles. The children would not have had these troubles had they not first had measles.

Necessity of care in measles

If you have measles, do not let others come near you, and do not think that, because you do not feel very sick, you can run about as usual. If you do not take good care of yourself, you may have some of the diseases that so often begin when children are getting over measles. Measles causes more deaths than is commonly supposed, especially among young children and very old people; and a great many children die of diseases which they never would have had if they had not first had the measles. Avoid people who have measles, and if you should get the disease, do not treat it as a slight thing, but consult your doctor at once.

Whooping Cough	*Scarlet Fever*	*Measles*	*Smallpox*
4,856	*4,309*	*4,302*	*74*

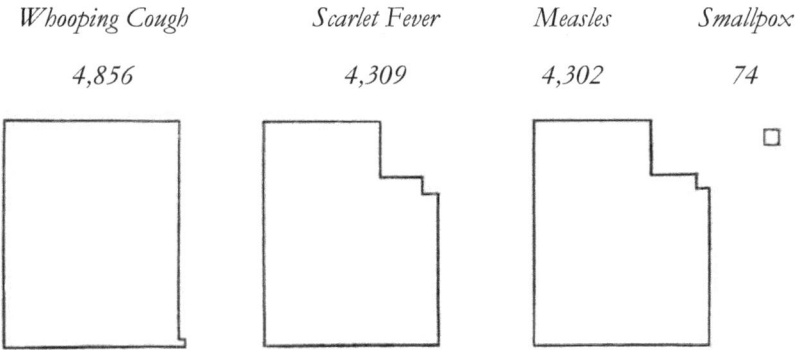

FIG. 61. Deaths in 1907 from four common communicable diseases reported to the United States Census Bureau.

Evil effects of whooping cough

Whooping cough is much the same as measles in this respect. It kills many children, and, in cases where it does not kill them, their bodies become so weakened that they are liable to contract some other disease that may prove fatal. Avoid people who have whooping cough.

Questions. 1. Why should people avoid measles? 2. Why should one take care of himself when he has measles? 3. Why is whooping cough to be avoided?

Remember. 1. Measles is more fatal, especially among babies, than people realize. 2. Measles causes more diseases of the bones, ears, and eyes than any other communicable disease. 3. Measles is not dangerous if properly cared for, but when neglected, it causes much suffering and many deaths. 4. Whooping cough causes almost as many deaths as does measles.

CHAPTER XXIX

HOW SMALLPOX IS PREVENTED

We now come to the study of a disease, the cause of which has not been positively recognized. We know that it is very communicable; but we know also that there is absolutely no reason for anyone's ever contracting it, since there is a way by which it may easily be prevented.

Fatality of smallpox before the discovery of vaccination

Something over a hundred years ago, smallpox was one of the most fatal diseases known. It is estimated that during the eighteenth century it killed over 60,000,000 people.

Up to the time when the Spaniards invaded Mexico, there had been no smallpox there. The Spaniards brought the disease with them, and historians tell us that out of the 12,000,000 people living in Mexico at that time, at least 6,000,000 died from smallpox. At that time the disease was considered fatal throughout the world; when it broke out in a community, people fled without stopping to bury their dead. It was a rare thing to see a person not more or less disfigured by the marks the disease leaves on the face and body.

To-day we find a very different condition. There are now fewer fatalities from smallpox than from almost any other communicable disease. During 1906 and 1907 only 169 deaths from smallpox were reported from all over the United States to the Census Bureau at Washington. What has caused this marked falling off in the fatality of the disease?

Discovery of vaccination

During the time that smallpox was killing so many people, all the doctors were trying to find something that would cure the disease or that would prevent it. In the latter part of the eighteenth century Dr. Edward Jenner, an English physician, noticed that milkmaids did not have smallpox as much as did people of other occupations. He also noticed cows with little sores on their udders that looked very much like the sores that come with smallpox. He therefore tried making on the arms of people sores just like those on the udders of the cows. He did this by taking a little of the matter from the sores on the cows and putting it into the scratches on the people's arms. After these sores had healed, the people who had been thus treated did not have smallpox. This simple practice has caused one of the most deadly diseases known to man to become one of the most easily controlled.

Prevention of smallpox by vaccination:

Though it is well known that before the discovery of vaccination smallpox was a fatal disease, there are still some persons who say that vaccination has done nothing to reduce the mortality. When you learn some of the facts, you can judge for yourself whether or not vaccination does prevent smallpox.

(1) In the Franco-Prussian War

During the Franco-Prussian War in 1870-71, the German soldiers were all vaccinated, and only a part of the French army was vaccinated. Smallpox broke out in the two armies. As a result, 6,000 of the French died from smallpox and only 278 of the Germans. In many instances, the German and the French soldiers were confined in the same hospitals, with exactly the same opportunities to contract the disease. But, you might ask, if vaccination prevents smallpox, how did it happen that there were *any* cases among the German soldiers? In order to prevent smallpox, vaccination must be successful; that is, it must "take." We will tell you about different kinds of vaccination a little later.

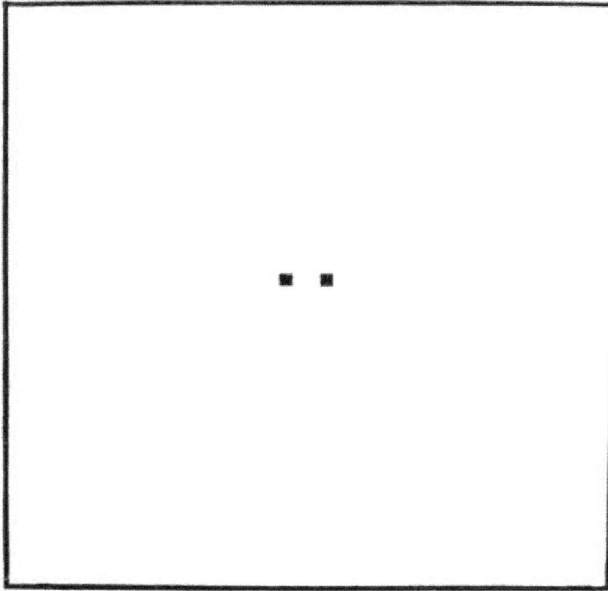

FIG. 62. In Sweden, before vaccination, smallpox caused 2,050 deaths per million population (represented by the large square). Since the introduction of vaccination the death rate has dropped to 2 per million population (represented by the two small squares).

(2) In Sweden

In Sweden we find strong evidence that vaccination prevents smallpox. Up to 1801, before vaccination was introduced into that country, the yearly death rate from smallpox was 2,050 out of each million of the population. In 1801 vaccination was introduced into Sweden, but the people were allowed to be vaccinated or not, just as they pleased. During the ten years ending with 1811, the annual death rate from smallpox had dropped from 2,050 per million of the population to 686 per million. Later, vaccination was made compulsory (that is, everybody in Sweden was obliged to be vaccinated), and in 1894 the death rate had dropped to only two deaths a year per million population. Is it merely a coincidence that this great falling off in deaths from smallpox came after vaccination was discovered, or was it due to vaccination?

(3) In the Philippine Islands

Before the Philippine Islands were occupied by the Americans, vaccination was very little practiced, and a large percentage of the deaths in those islands was caused by smallpox. In 1897 smallpox caused about 40,000 deaths. A few years later the Americans enforced vaccination among the inhabitants of the Philippines, and the result was that in 1907 there were only 304 deaths from smallpox. There has been practically no quarantine for smallpox and no disinfection; the only cause of the suppression of the disease in the Philippine Islands is vaccination—nothing else.

(4) In Gloucester, England

In Gloucester, England, there used to be a great many people who did not believe in vaccination, though it is doubtful if they themselves could have explained why they did not. They seem to have been much like the man who, when asked, "What do you think of this?" replied, "I don't know anything about it, but I am against it." In 1890 Gloucester had a population of 42,000 people, most of whom had never been vaccinated. In the latter part of 1895, smallpox broke out. Quarantine was strictly carried out, but the disease continued to spread. As the people saw the number of victims rapidly increasing, many of them concluded that they had rather be vaccinated than have smallpox, even though they did not really believe in vaccination. By the first of April, 1896, over 36,000 people had been vaccinated in Gloucester, and by the first of August there was not a case of smallpox in the city. But what had happened in the meantime? There had been 1,979 cases of smallpox; a very large amount of money had been expended in quarantining; hundreds of persons had been disfigured for life; and 439 lives had been lost. And all this simply because the people did not believe in vaccination.

Quarantining smallpox is a most expensive luxury, which may possibly retard the progress of this disease, but was never known to check an epidemic of it. Every epidemic of smallpox during the last one hundred years has been checked by vaccination.

Why some diseases do not return

There are certain diseases which you are not likely to have more than once; one attack protects against another. Why and how does one attack of a certain disease protect against another? When a person is taken sick with one of these diseases, the cells of his body immediately begin to make a substance called antitoxin. We learned something about antitoxin when we were studying diphtheria. In diseases like scarlet fever, measles, and smallpox, in which one attack protects against another, the antitoxin that is formed in the body when you are sick stays there for a long time, in some cases as long as you live. While this antitoxin is present in the blood, the cause of the disease cannot live in the body; hence you cannot have the disease again. After some diseases this antitoxin seems to disappear from the blood in a short time; after others, it seems to remain for several years; and after still others it remains as long as you live. After diphtheria it stays in the blood only a short time, so that one may have diphtheria a second time within a few years. Some people have smallpox, measles, or scarlet fever a second time, but with most people these diseases never return.

If we knew how to make the cells of our bodies produce this antitoxin and keep it stored up in the blood all the time, we should never have any of these diseases. But in many cases we do not know how to cause the cells to manufacture this antitoxin. However, in one or two diseases we do know how to persuade them to make the antitoxin, and the one in which we know how to accomplish this best is smallpox. This is just what is done by vaccination.

How vaccination prevents smallpox

The object of vaccination is to put the cells of the body to work making antitoxin. To do this, it is necessary to get some of the toxin into the body. We want to get in just enough to make the cells work, and no more. Therefore we make a very small scratch, and put into it some of the vaccine which contains the toxin of smallpox. It is impossible to have these germs in your body and not be affected by them to some degree. If you did not feel a little sick, the cells would not be making antitoxin, for the thing that makes you sick is what makes the cells go to work. But this sickness is only a matter of a day or two, and after the cells have made the antitoxin, it will stay in your body a long time, longer in some cases than in others.

Some people, after they have once been vaccinated, can never be successfully vaccinated again; neither can such people ever have smallpox. Most people, however, can be successfully vaccinated every five to seven years, and there are a few people who will "take" if vaccinated every year or two. These conditions indicate the length of time that the antitoxin of smallpox will live in the bodies of these different persons. If vaccination, properly performed, does not take, the person is not in a condition at that time to catch smallpox; and if vaccination, properly performed, does take, it is positive evidence that if this person had been exposed to smallpox, he would have taken the disease.

Necessity of repeated vaccination

It is frequently asked, "How long will vaccination protect against smallpox?" You can no more answer this question than you can tell how long the antitoxin will live in the blood of any particular person. The only safe thing to do is to be vaccinated every few years, and if smallpox is present in your community, get vaccinated every year until the vaccination takes. If it takes, it shows that you were in a condition to catch the disease; and if it does not take, you may feel safe from smallpox for a while, at least.

Questions. 1. Why was smallpox formerly more widespread and more often fatal than it is now? 2. Tell of the discovery of vaccination. 3. Give instances to show the influence of vaccination on smallpox epidemics. 4. Why must there be repeated vaccinations? 5. Show how vaccinating for smallpox is like taking antitoxin to prevent diphtheria.

Remember. 1. Before the introduction of vaccination, smallpox was one of the most dangerous diseases known. 2. All evidence of history tends to show that vaccination has caused smallpox to become a very mild disease and a comparatively rare one. 3. Successful vaccination repeated at proper intervals will prevent smallpox. 4. Vaccination must be repeated because we do not know just how long the material developed in the body from a single vaccination will last.

CHAPTER XXX

WHY VACCINATION SOMETIMES SEEMS A FAILURE

What constitutes a successful vaccination

How does it happen that those who have been recently vaccinated sometimes have smallpox? It is *successful* vaccination that prevents smallpox, not recent vaccination; there is a vast difference between the two. A *successful* vaccination is one that results in a sore identical with the sores of smallpox. Such a sore is secured only as a result of the action of the germs that cause smallpox.

If the arm is red from the shoulder to the wrist and so swollen that you cannot use it for weeks, it does not necessarily mean that you have had a successful vaccination.

Such arms are not the result of vaccination itself, any more than a railroad wreck is the result of the fact that there is steam in the engine. The railroad wreck is caused by carelessness on the part of some operator, and the badly inflamed and swollen arm is due to lack of care or knowledge on the part of the vaccinator or the person vaccinated.

Some pretended vaccinations

A fly blister is not a successful vaccination. Such a statement may not seem necessary, until you hear this story. A man showed a sore on his arm, asserting that it was a successful vaccination. He was told that it was nothing but the result of a blister, and not vaccination, and that the work had been done by putting a small bit of blistering plaster on his arm. He admitted this to be the fact, and said that the "doctor" who did it told him that it was a new way of vaccinating. The doctors who say that vaccination will not prevent smallpox belong to the class who use fly blisters and call them vaccinations. When the patient gets smallpox, those who are opposed to vaccinations say that here is an illustration of their claim that vaccination will not prevent smallpox.

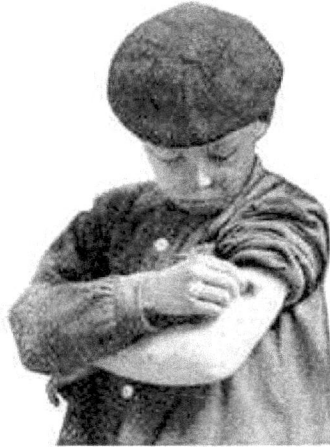

FIG. 63. How vaccinated arms are sometimes infected.

Some people who honestly think they were vaccinated have smallpox. There are sometimes instances in which a person recently vaccinated with apparent success nevertheless contracts smallpox; there are still other cases in which the disease develops after a vaccination that would not take. Here is an example:

A doctor vaccinates a child in the usual manner. At the end of four or five days, the dressing is taken from the arm, and the only thing to be seen is a little black scab. The child scratches this off. In a few days the spot becomes red and a small abscess forms, resembling a smallpox sore. Naturally, this is taken for a completely successful vaccination, but it is not really so. When the child scratched off the scab, the vaccination wound was nearly healed, and the little abscess was caused by some very mild pus germs, which were under the finger nails with which he scratched the wound. The abscess was in no wise connected with the vaccination, but was simply such an infection as a child might get at any time that he scratched his arm. No one has ever claimed that such an abscess will prevent smallpox any more than that a boil will prevent it.

A successful vaccination will prevent smallpox. The length of time for which it will prevent the disease varies in different individuals. Some it will protect only for a year or two, while in others it will last through life.

Dr. H. W. Bond, Health Commissioner of St. Louis, Missouri, states:

"The experience of this department, based on the observation of thousands of cases, is that a well-pitted mark gives at least ten years' immunity. We have never seen a case of smallpox in a person with a well-pitted scar less than ten years old—that is, the scar less than ten years old."

A sore arm not always due to successful vaccination

One of the strongest objections made against vaccination is that the arm sometimes becomes very sore from it. This is true, but the sore arm is not a common occurrence and is never caused by vaccination properly performed. There is always some cause for the bad arm besides the vaccination.

Cause of sore arms

The usual cause of a bad arm is improper vaccination; this means the lack of proper precautions on the part of the person who does the vaccinating. Years ago, before vaccination was performed with the great care which is given it to-day, bad arms could not be prevented; but to-day the cause of the trouble is not the vaccine, but the vaccinator. Sometimes a father thinks he will save a dollar by vaccinating his child himself, and he is likely to injure the child by attempting to vaccinate him without taking antiseptic precautions. The same surgical preparations must be made for a vaccination as for an operation. If this is not done, a bad arm will result, not because of the vaccination, but because of the negligence of the vaccinator.

Never allow any person, doctor or otherwise, to vaccinate you until the skin surface has been well washed with soap and water, rinsed clean, and wiped off with alcohol. See that the vaccine is fresh and has been properly kept. When it begins to "take," keep the spot absolutely clean and covered with a clean cloth, renewed daily. *Never scratch or rub it.* These precautions will prevent the dreaded soreness of the arm.

How people themselves infect their arms with pus germs

The person operated on is himself often responsible for the bad arm. A careful doctor will put a dressing on the arm, after he has supplied the vaccine, and will tell you to let that dressing alone, for he wishes to take it off himself. About the third or fourth day after the vaccination, your arm begins to itch. Possibly you have forgotten what the doctor told you; at any rate, you pay no attention to directions and take the dressing off to scratch the arm. When you scratch the wound, you introduce pus germs into it, and you have no reason to expect anything but a sore arm. In this case, it is not the fault of the vaccinator or of the vaccination; it is your own fault. Never touch a vaccination sore; in fact, it is dangerous to touch any sore.

Questions. 1. How is a successful vaccination determined? 2. What are some pretended vaccinations? 3. Mention some of the things that cause bad arms after vaccination.

Remember. 1. A successful vaccination causes a sore identical with the sores that result from smallpox. 2. A fly blister is not a vaccination in any sense of the word. 3. A very sore arm does not result from a properly performed vaccination, but from carelessness on the part of the vaccinator or the person vaccinated.

CHAPTER XXXI

CONSUMPTION, THE GREAT WHITE PLAGUE

Tuberculosis, or consumption, has been known for many centuries. It was known long before Rome was ever heard of. Hippocrates, a Greek physician, studied it, and said that if it were treated in its early stages, it could be cured.

Why consumption is called the Great White Plague

Tuberculosis is called the Great White Plague. It is called the Great Plague, because it kills more people than does any other one disease; the White Plague, because people who suffer from it become so pale and white.

Consumption more destructive than war

It is estimated that nearly 200,000 people die from tuberculosis every year in the United States. This means that in this country there is one death from consumption every two minutes and thirty-six seconds. Is it not fearful to think of nearly 200,000 people dying every year, in the United States alone, from a disease that we know can be prevented? Do you not think that we ought to do everything we can to prevent this disease from spreading?

During the Civil War 205,070 soldiers were killed in both armies. This war lasted four years. During the same length of time there were 640,000 deaths from tuberculosis in the United States. This means that consumption killed over three times as many people as were killed during the same length of time in the Civil War. In some parts of the country one out of every seven deaths is caused by this disease, but the average throughout the country is one death out of every ten.

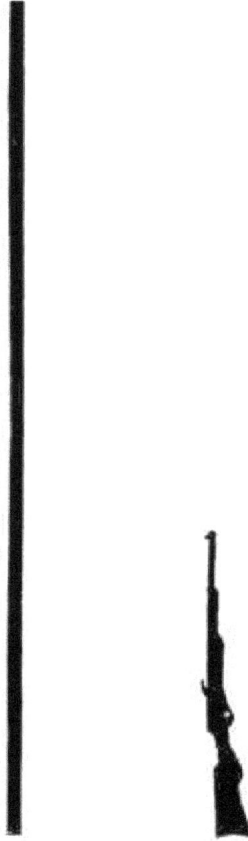

FIG. 64. Comparing 640,000 deaths from tuberculosis the United States during four years with the 205,070 deaths in the Civil War.

Prevalence of tuberculosis

There are more than 700,000 people sick from tuberculosis every year in the United States alone. Of this number nearly 200,000 die every year. Tuberculosis is a disease that can be prevented. It may take a long time to get rid of it, but it can be abolished. When you think of all the people that are sick from tuberculosis, and of all those who die from it every year, you will surely want to do all you can to help prevent this suffering and death.

Tuberculosis a disease of various parts of the body:

When people speak of consumption they usually mean tuberculosis of the lungs; but tuberculosis is not confined to the lungs. The germs that cause tuberculosis may attack any part of the body, and from one part may go to other parts, setting up a growth wherever they go.

(1) Of the throat

Tuberculosis of the throat is a common form of the disease. When the germs of tuberculosis settle in the throat, they destroy the tissues very rapidly and, as a rule, kill the patient much more quickly than they do when they start in the lungs.

(2) Of the joints

Another frequent form of tuberculosis in occurs in the knee; this is popularly called "white swelling." It quickly destroys the knee joint and results in a stiff leg. The growth may stop there, but more often it extends from the knee to other parts of the body.

Often we see a little boy or girl wearing one shoe with a sole much thicker than the other. This is because one leg is shorter than the other, and we notice that the shortened leg is deformed as well. This condition sometimes results from an injury, but it is far more likely to be caused by tuberculosis of the hip joint.

(3) Of the spine

Again we see boys and girls with diseases of the spine, so that they have "hunch backs" or are twisted to one side. These conditions result from tuberculosis of the bones of the spine.

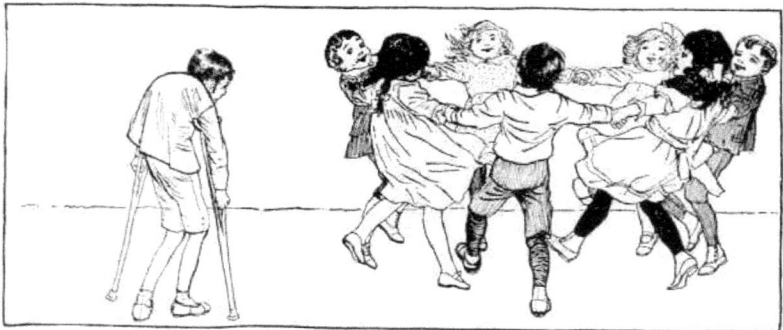

FIG. 65. One of the effects of tuberculosis.

(4) Of the glands

Sometimes we see children and grown people with swellings on their necks. These swellings may look smooth, but they feel as if they were made up of little bunches of grapes or plums under the skin. They are almost always due to the growth of the germs that cause tuberculosis of the little glands of the neck.

(5) Of the stomach

Any one of the other glands of the body is just as liable to become affected by tuberculosis as are the glands of the neck. Tuberculosis of the stomach or bowels is not at all uncommon.

The germs of tuberculosis are likely to attack any of the tissues of the body, especially if the cells composing these tissues are for any reason weakened so that they cannot do the work required of them. When the tuberculosis germs grow in tissues, the tissues finally break down and an abscess forms. A tubercular abscess is sometimes called a "cold abscess."

All such abscesses finally break and an open sore results. The matter that comes from the open sore and from the abscess when it is first opened is full of the germs that cause tuberculosis. If this matter is allowed to become dry, the germs are blown about in the dust. Then other people may inhale them or take them into their bodies through the mouth or skin and thus contract consumption.

The old belief that consumption is inherited

Until a few years ago it was generally believed that consumption was inherited. That is, it was thought that children whose father or mother had consumption were born with the disease. Even to-day many people hold to this idea, because they have not studied or learned of the discoveries made in recent years. These people still believe that if a child's father or mother dies of tuberculosis, the child will die of tuberculosis, too, no matter how careful he may be or how much of a fight he may make against it.

It is true that many people whose parents have died of consumption also die from this disease; but this does not prove that they were born with consumption. It merely shows that they had a good chance to catch the disease by being continually with some one who had it. It is also true that a great many people die from consumption whose parents did not have it. If consumption is an inherited disease, where did these people get it?

About thirty years ago, Dr. Robert Koch discovered that all consumptives have in their sputum a long, slender germ which he called the tubercle bacillus. Some of these germs he injected into guinea pigs, and he found that they caused the pigs to have consumption. Then he made many other experiments, and proved beyond question that it is this very germ that causes tuberculosis, and that no one has consumption unless he has this germ in his body.

Evidence that consumption is not inherited

Then the question arose, "Is the baby whose parents have consumption born with this germ in its body?" This question could not at first be answered; but tests were made by taking the children of consumptive parents away from their parents, and keeping them in homes where there were no consumptives. It was found that these babies did not develop the disease. From these and many other tests, it has been proved that consumption is not inherited, and that the reason the child of the consumptive so often has consumption is because he lives with people having the disease.

Evidence that consumption is a house disease

Consumption seems to be confined to certain families, and this has led many people to think that the disease is inherited, regardless of the proof that it is not. When we carefully study the facts in various cases, we find that the disease is not confined to a certain family, so much as it is to the *house* in which the family lives.

The record of a single house will illustrate how tuberculosis sticks to the house rather than to the family. From 1880 to 1901, a particular house was occupied by a father, mother, and six children, of whom four died of consumption. From 1902 to 1903 the house was occupied by another father and mother with eight children. They moved away because of the great amount of sickness in the family. At present this father and one of his children have tuberculosis. In 1904 the house was occupied by still another family, consisting likewise of a father, mother, and eight children. Now it is known that four of the children have tuberculosis, and it is feared that three others have also contracted the disease. In 1905 a son of the first occupant, with his wife and two children, returned to live in the house. The father of this family died of tuberculosis. Up to 1906 the total results from this house, scattered through four families, were as follows: five deaths, six cases in people still living, and three suspected cases.

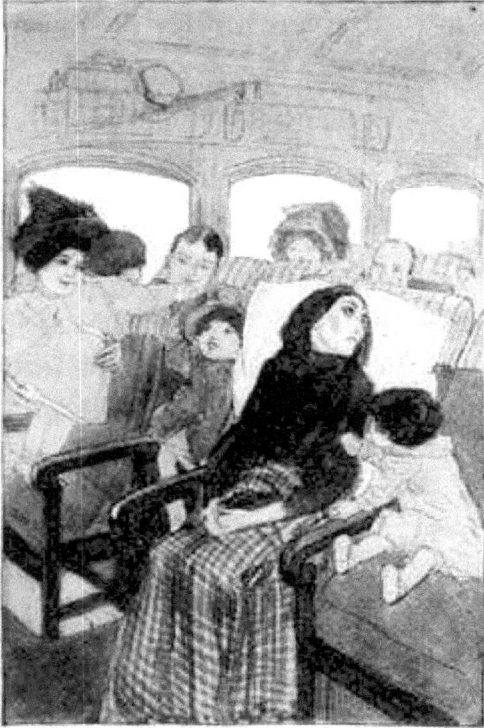

FIG. 66. The constant danger of infection in railway cars, where germs can live as well as in a house.

Why consumption is a house disease

When the consumptive coughs, he sends fine droplets of moisture into the air. These droplets contain the germs that cause tuberculosis. The moisture evaporates and the germs are left sticking to the floors, the walls, the curtains, and the furniture of the room. When the room is swept or dusted, the germs are stirred up with the dust and people inhale them. The germ that causes consumption will live for a long time in a house; you cannot see it, but it is there. Wherever a consumptive has lived, he has left the germs of this disease behind him.

How to disinfect houses

If a house in which a consumptive has lived is thoroughly disinfected, all the germs he left there will be killed. Scattering disinfectants about a room does no good. The only proper way to disinfect is to close the house, for if the disinfectant is strong enough to kill the disease germs, no human being can stay in the house while it is being used. Disinfecting should be done by the health officer, because he knows how much disinfectant is needed to kill every germ in the house and how it should be used.

Fraudulent disinfectants

Sometimes you will see an advertisement saying that certain disinfectants will kill the germs of disease but will not affect the people. Always remember that any disinfectant that is strong enough to kill the disease germs will also kill human beings, and do not be fooled by such advertisements.

Never move into a house that has been previously occupied, until the house has been disinfected. Do not take it for granted that the people who lived there before had no communicable disease. Do not take the word of the agent or of any one else that there has never been sickness in the house. People sometimes have tuberculosis without knowing it; people sometimes have tuberculosis or other communicable diseases without telling of it.

It does not cost much to disinfect a house, and if the disinfection is properly done the disease germs will be killed. "An ounce of prevention is worth a pound of cure." Try to convince your father that by having the new home disinfected he may save not only doctor's fees, but perhaps the lives of himself and his family.

There are a great many things that boys and girls can do to help fight this disease. This "scourge" can be wiped out; but if the boys and girls do not help in this great work, it will never be done.

Questions. 1. Why do people call consumption the Great White Plague? 2. What is the annual death rate from consumption in the United States? 3. Compare the fatality from consumption with the number of soldiers killed during the Civil War. 4. What amount of illness in the United States is due to consumption? 5. Describe at least four forms of tuberculosis. 6. What determines the part of the body in which the germ of tuberculosis grows?

Remember. 1. Tuberculosis and consumption are the same disease. 2. This disease kills more people than war, although it might be prevented. 3. Tuberculosis is not confined to the lungs but may attack the tissues of any part of the body. 4. Consumption is not inherited; it is a house disease rather than a family disease. 5. A house should be disinfected by the health officer before it is occupied by a new tenant.

CHAPTER XXXII

HOW CONSUMPTION IS SPREAD AND HOW PREVENTED

The sputum (spit) of the consumptive and the discharges from tubercular sores contain the germs that cause tuberculosis. Sometimes these germs are so numerous that thousands of them would be found clinging to the point of a needle dipped into the sputum or discharges from a patient. When the consumptive coughs, he sends into the air many of the germs that cause tuberculosis.

We cannot kill the germs while they are in the body of the consumptive; but we can kill them after they have left the body, by seeing that none of the sputum or discharge from tubercular wounds or sores is allowed to become dried and blown about as dust.

(1) In discharges from sores

When the discharge from a tubercular sore becomes dried and blows about with the dust, the germs are inhaled into the lungs of other people, or fall into other sores and cause them to become tubercular. Since this is one of the most frequent ways by which this dread disease is spread, you will say at once, "Why, every particle of matter from a tubercular sore ought to be burned, so that there would be no possibility of the germs being scattered." This of course ought to be done, but this is not enough.

People sometimes have consumption and are not aware that they have it. Others may have tubercular sores and not know them to be such. Any sore, whether it is tubercular or not, contains disease germs. They may not be the germs of tuberculosis, but even the least dangerous of them is the germ that causes pus (matter).

Since we are trying to get rid not only of the germs that cause tuberculosis, but also of the germs that cause all communicable diseases, it would be better to say, "All discharges from *any* sore should be burned immediately."

(2) In the sputum

When people spit on the sidewalk or on the floor, the sputum will of course become dry. Sometimes a lady drags her dress through the sputum on the sidewalk or on the floor; it sticks to her dress and she takes the germs home with her. The sputum of the consumptive is loaded with the germs that cause tuberculosis, and if this sputum is allowed to be blown about with the dust, people will inhale it and thus get the germs into their lungs. Certainly the consumptive should never spit on the sidewalk or on the floor, or in the mine, workshop, or in any place where the sputum may become dry and form dust. Of course he should not fill the air about him with germs by coughing into it; everybody knows that.

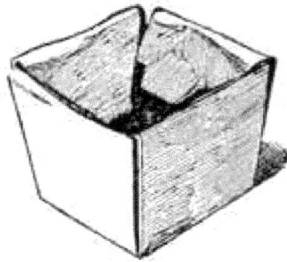

FIG. 67. A sputum cup of waterproof pasteboard.

Why everybody should be careful about spitting and coughing

But *no* man or woman, boy or girl, should ever spit on the floor or sidewalk. In the first place it is bad manners. No person does this who is well brought up. In the second place, we must remember that the consumptive does not like to have others know that he has consumption; this feeling is a part of the disease. If you expect the consumptive to refrain from spitting on the floor or sidewalk, you must help him by your example. You cannot expect him to be the only one to hunt up a cuspidor, when you yourself are spitting on floor or sidewalk. If you expect the consumptive to take the precaution necessary to protect you from this disease, you must take the same precaution yourself.

In the matter of coughing, the same rules hold true. If you expect the consumptive to hold a handkerchief before his mouth when he coughs, you must do the same.

How to avoid spitting on the floor or sidewalk:

Since it is not right that the consumptive should spit on the floor or sidewalk, it will naturally be asked, "What is the consumptive to do with what he coughs up?"

(1) By using paper napkins

At a very small cost he can buy paper napkins and envelopes which have been treated with paraffin to prevent moisture going through them. If every one with a cough or with any such trouble as catarrh, which makes him want to spit frequently, would carry a supply of these paper napkins and paraffin envelopes, he would always have a suitable place in which to spit. When you cough up anything, spit into one of these little napkins, put the napkin into the envelope, and when you get home burn the whole thing.

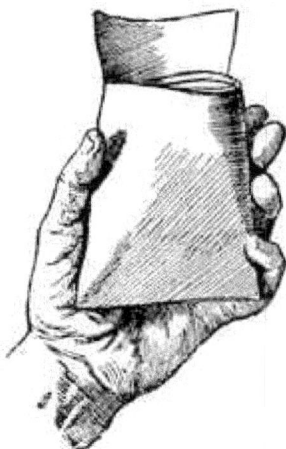

FIG. 68. A pocket cuspidor.

(2) By using pocket cuspidors

There are other conveniences which can easily be carried in the pocket, called pocket cuspidors. Some are made of thin cardboard, treated with paraffin, and filled with cotton to hold all the moisture of the sputum; others are made of glass, shaped like a bottle, with a wide mouth. Those made of cardboard should be burned as soon as possible and the glass ones should be thoroughly washed with boiling water.

(3) By having public cuspidors

In some cities cuspidors have been placed at the edge of the sidewalk in an effort to lessen the spread of disease caused by spitting. These cuspidors have a stream of water running through them constantly and are connected with the sewer. They are so made that they cannot easily be kicked over or upset, and they are placed on stands just high enough to make it easy to spit into them. If properly made, they are not unsightly. Would it not be a good thing if your town would put such cuspidors on your streets, and if the merchants would put them into their stores? Every office, every workshop, every store, every railway and street car should be provided with cuspidors.

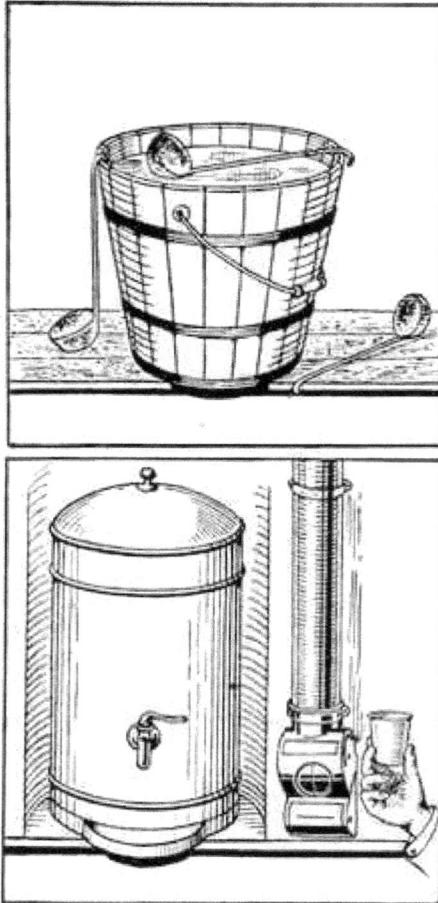

FIG. 69. The common drinking cup—a fruitful source of infection.

FIG. 70. The individual drinking cup—each cup clean and free from disease germs.

We know that the substance which people cough up when they have consumption contains the germs that cause this disease. When they spit this matter out, many of the germs stick to the lips. This is true not only of consumption, but of the germs of other diseases, such as diphtheria, measles, and scarlet fever.

(1) By drinking cups

When there are disease germs on the lips, it is impossible for a person to drink and not leave some of the germs sticking to the edge of the cup or glass. If the germs of disease are in the mouth, every time that the person suffering from this disease drinks from a cup, he leaves some of the germs on the edge of it. The next person to drink from that cup may get the germs into his mouth.

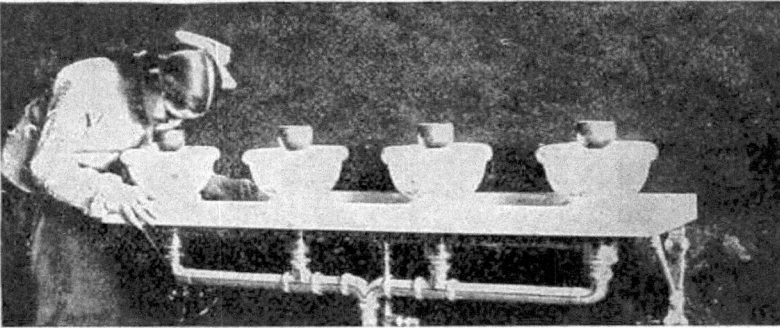

FIG. 71. A sanitary drinking fountain for public places.

Always avoid drinking from a cup or glass from which another person has been drinking. You can never tell who may have disease germs in his mouth, or when you may get them on your lips by drinking from the same cup. Each individual should have his own cup and should never let any one else drink from it.

(2) By putting pencils into the mouth

When you put the point of your pencil into your mouth, you will leave germs on it just as you do on the edge of a cup when you drink. Never put your pencil into your mouth; never use any other person's pencil; never trade pencils.

Sometimes we see a child giving his friends a bite of his apple or candy or cake. Of course when disease germs are in the mouth of the one who takes a bite, the germs will be left on the apple, candy, or cake. By no means should a boy or girl be selfish, but if you have something to share with your friends, break it or cut it into pieces. Never take into your mouth anything from which another person has taken a bite.

How tubercular cows cause consumption

Milk that comes from consumptive cows may contain the germs that cause tuberculosis. When you drink the milk from such cows, you take these germs into your body. They find their way from the stomach and intestine into the blood, and there they travel about until they find a spot where the cells are dead or are not doing their work properly. When they find such a place, they settle down and begin to grow; and the first thing you know, you will have tuberculosis in that part of your body. Sometimes the germs do not have to go out of the stomach or intestines to find a favorable opportunity to take hold and grow. When this happens, we have consumption of the bowels.

One cannot tell by looking at milk or by tasting it whether or not the germs of tuberculosis are present. They do not make the milk sour; neither do they make it look different from pure milk.

One cannot tell by looking at a cow whether or not she has tuberculosis. Sometimes a cow will have tuberculosis and yet look very healthy. There is, however, a way by which we can tell when a cow has this disease, no matter how healthy she may look. This is what is known as the tuberculin test.

How to detect tuberculosis in a cow

If a little tuberculin is injected under the skin of a cow that has tuberculosis, it will make her have a fever and appear sick for a day or two. If she is free from tuberculosis, it will not make her sick at all.

It would seem as if all people who sell milk would want to know whether their cows have consumption so as not to run any risk of conveying the disease to their customers. Some of them do take this precaution, but a great many of them do not want to go to this trouble. Sometimes you will hear them say, "Oh, I do not believe in this tuberculin test." They do not want to believe in it because they know that the cows, if tested and found to have tuberculosis, will have to be killed.

The reason that dairymen sell us milk from tubercular cows is the same that makes the man with scarlet fever in his house fail to tell the health officer about it; the same that makes the butcher buy and sell meat from diseased cattle; the same that makes some people absolutely regardless of the welfare of others—it is selfishness.

Questions. 1. How does a patient give off tuberculosis germs? 2. Why should even well people refrain from spitting in public? 3. Why should the sputum be taken care of? 4. Why should we avoid the common drinking cup? 5. What is the danger from putting pencils into the mouth? 6. Is it safe to use another person's pencil? 7. What is the best way of sharing food? 8. How can one be protected from tubercular milk?

Remember. 1. The sputum and discharges from all sores should be immediately burned or disposed of in such a way that they cannot become dry and be blown about as dust. 2. Consumption may be contracted by the use of the common drinking cup, or by putting into your mouth such things as pencils and coins. 3. The milk from a cow suffering from consumption contains the germ of tuberculosis. 4. A cow may have tuberculosis and not appear to be sick. 5. The only way to determine whether a cow has tuberculosis is by using the tuberculin test. 6. Every milch cow should be tuberculin tested.

———————————————————————————————

CHAPTER XXXIII

HOW CONSUMPTION IS CURED

Consumption should be recognized early

When people first get consumption, they seldom realize that they are seriously sick. Most of them think they have a bad cold, or are overworked, or that they have been staying too closely in the house. Often they will not even see a doctor until they are so sick that the doctor cannot do much for them.

When you have a slight cough that "hangs on"; when you feel feverish every afternoon; when you are short of breath; when you get tired very easily; when you do not feel like eating anything except candies and cakes— then you should think of consumption. These are not all the signs, but they are enough to make you go at once to a doctor.

A long time ago the doctor would have felt badly if he had been obliged to tell you that you had consumption; but now he knows that if you go to him early in the disease and follow his directions, you will get well.

How consumption is cured: (1) By rest

When the doctor finds that a person has consumption, the first thing he orders is rest. By this he means absolute *rest*. He does not mean that the patient can go to school or to the office part of the day and rest the remainder of the day. The doctor will want to watch him constantly. Then there comes a time when he must begin to take a little exercise; the doctor tells him just how much exercise to take, and just what form of exercise is best for him.

(2) By fresh air

The consumptive must have plenty of fresh air all the time; he must be out-of-doors as much as possible. You will wonder how the doctor expects him to be out-of-doors when he has been told that he must have absolute rest. Later we will show you how one can practically be out-of-doors and yet at the same time be in bed.

(3) By sunshine

Sunshine will kill the germs of any disease more quickly than almost anything we know of, and a consumptive must have all the sunshine that he can get. Of course it cannot get into the body to kill the germs, but it strengthens the cells of the body so much that they can fight with just that much more energy.

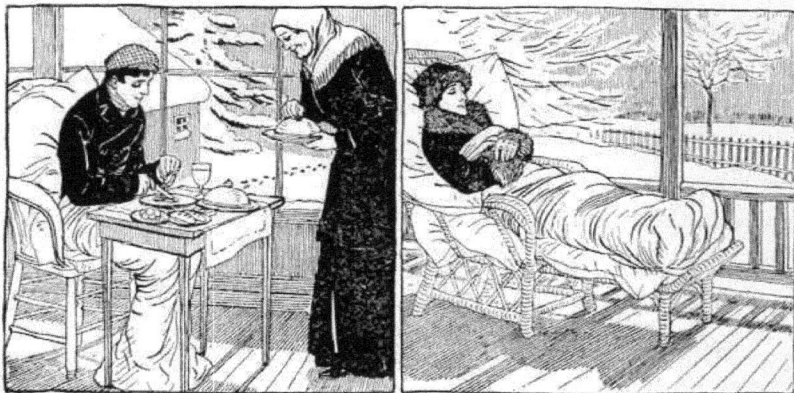

FIGS. 72 and 73. Living outdoors in cold weather.

(4) By nourishing food

Nothing is more important than pure food in building up the body and in making heat and power. In consumption the food that is stored up in the body burns itself up very fast. The consumptive must therefore take not only the food needed to supply the usual demands of the body, but enough to make something extra for the disease to burn up without drawing on the reserve fund stored in the body. In order to do this, he will have to eat a great deal, and what he eats must be of the kind that makes the best building material and the most nourishing material. He cannot tax his stomach by eating things that are not nourishing; all the work his stomach can do must be devoted to the foods he really needs.

The weapons with which we fight consumption are rest, good food, fresh air, and sunshine. These will do more good than all the medicine in the world. Fresh air is not only one of the best things for the cure of consumption, but it is one of the best things for the prevention of consumption. You should always breathe plenty of fresh air night and day, and there is plenty of fresh air to be had if you will take it.

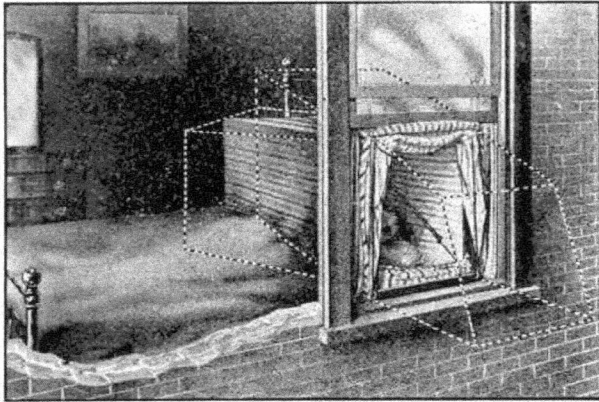

FIG. 74. A window tent. (Invented by Dr. W. E. Walsh.)

How to have fresh air at home:

If you have only a single window in your room, try to sleep with your head in the fresh air. It is not always easy to arrange a room in such a way that you can have fresh air without placing your bed in a draft, but even this difficulty can be overcome.

(1) By window tents

There are several devices, called window tents, which you can buy. By the use of such a tent, your head will be out-of-doors all the time; yet the draft cannot strike your body, because a part of the tent fits around your neck and cuts off the air from the rest of your body. One of these tents is shown in Figure 74. You do not put your head out of the window; your head is on your pillow just as if the tent were not there. Your bed is placed directly in front of the window and the tent comes down over your pillow, allowing your head practically to be out-of-doors, but keeping the cold air out of the room. Sleeping under a window tent is the next best thing to sleeping out-of-doors.

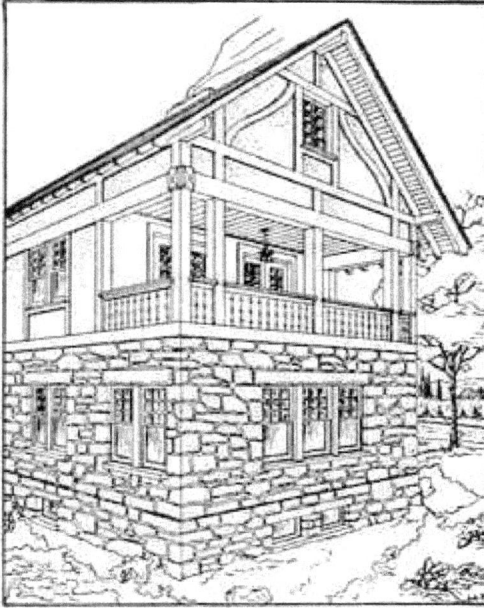

FIG. 75. A sleeping porch built in a house.

(2) By sleeping porches

Many of our modern houses are built with sleeping porches on which one can sleep outdoors summer and winter. Where there is not a special sleeping porch on the house, an ordinary porch may often be made to serve the purpose, or a very inexpensive sleeping porch can be added to the house.

(3) By tent cots

Sometimes people cannot get the use of a porch of any kind. In such cases it may be possible to put up a tent in the yard. If the yard is very small, a tent cot may be used. This is simply a cot with a tent on it, which can be closed up and put away in the daytime and set up again at night. In a large city where the houses have no yards at all, this arrangement can be used by setting it up on the roof of the house. There is almost always some way of securing fresh air at night if we will only give a little thought to the matter.

Fresh air in schoolrooms

Unfortunately, many of our school buildings are not provided with good ventilating plants. A proper system of ventilation furnishes at least 1200 cubic feet of fresh air per hour for each child in each room.

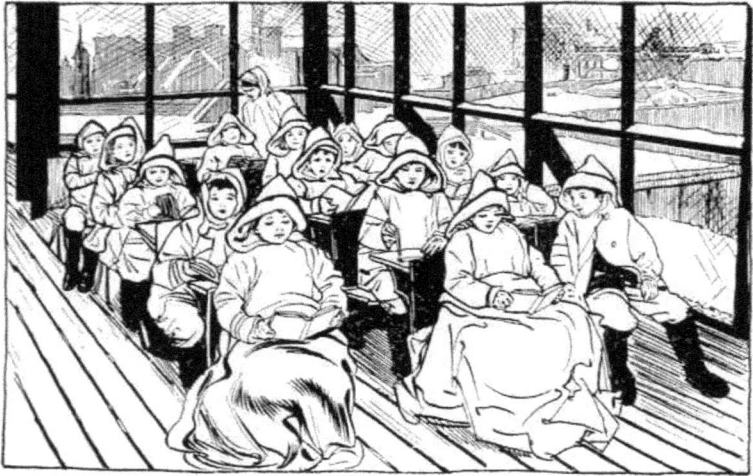

FIG. 76. An open-air schoolroom for consumptive children.

The necessity for playgrounds

In large cities it is often impossible to find outdoor space in which boys and girls may play during recess. Even this difficulty can be overcome by turning the roof of the school building into a playground, with a high wire netting around it.

Every school yard should be provided with swings, bars, and gymnasium apparatus to encourage the children to take plenty of exercise. Children who live in crowded towns need exercise during vacation as well as during school days, and the school yards should be open to them at all times. A summer teacher who shows the children the best way to exercise, has work fully as important as that of any other teacher during the school term.

A sound body is more valuable than education itself, but a good education and a sound body together are the best assets any man or woman can have.

Questions. 1. State the four things necessary to cure consumption; show the value of each. 2. What is the value of fresh air to every one? 3. How may an abundance of fresh air be secured in the home? 4. In the school?

Remember. 1. Rest, fresh air, sunshine, and nourishing food are the cures for consumption. 2. All these things can be secured in any climate and by every person. 3. **Tuberculosis is a communicable disease.** 4. **Tuberculosis can be prevented.** 5. **Tuberculosis can be cured.**

APPENDIX

A SUMMARY OF ANATOMY

BONES AND JOINTS

The framework of the body

The framework of the body is composed of bones. There are 206 bones (not including the teeth) in the body. The bones of the body are divided into four classes—long bones, short bones, flat bones, and irregular bones.

Construction of bones

Regardless of their shape, all bones are composed in the same way. Every bone has an outer and an inner portion. The outer portion is a dense layer called *compact bone*. The inner portion is more open, and is much weaker; this is called *cancellated bone* (from *cancella*, a sponge). In the smaller bones, the marrow, which is quite soft, runs through the spongy bone; in the larger long bones, the marrow is distinct and is enclosed by the spongy bone.

The periosteum

Every bone is covered by a thick, tough layer, the *periosteum*, which has three uses. When the bone is injured by disease or accident, the periosteum makes new bone to fill in and repair the break. It also builds new bone on the surface of the old as long as the body is growing. Finally, the periosteum gives strong and firm attachment to the muscles, which send tendons into it.

Joints

Every bone in the body (except the hyoid bone, to which the tongue is attached) is joined with some other bone. Most of them join with two or more bones. In most instances the end of a bone which joins with another is rounded off and made very smooth, so that it can slide easily over the other bone. There are three principal kinds of joints in the body. They are called the *ball and socket* joint, the *hinge* joint, and the *serrated* or *saw-tooth* joint.

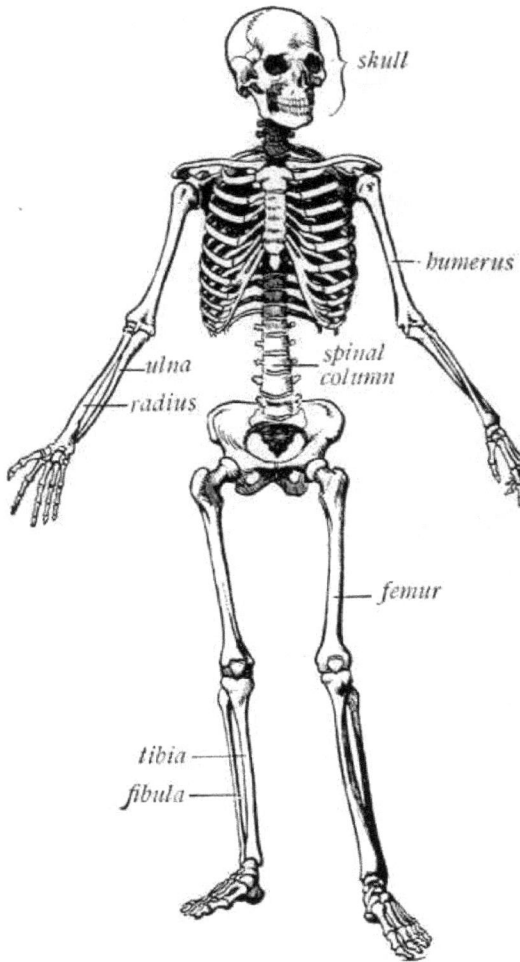

FIG. 77. The skeleton.

The ball and socket joint

The ball and socket joint is one that can move freely in all directions. We see it illustrated in the joints of the shoulder and hip. In these joints one of the bones has a deep depression in it, and this depression forms the *socket*. The other bone has a rounded head that fits into the depression. We call this rounded head the *ball*.

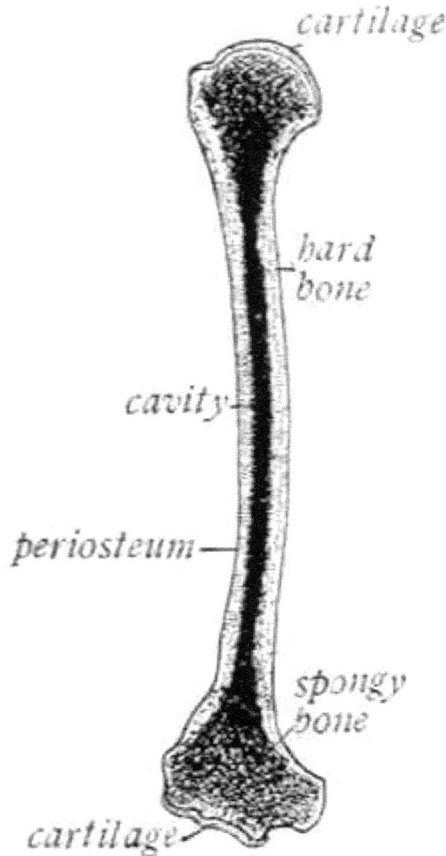

FIG. 78. The structure of a bone.

The hinge joint

The hinge joint is illustrated in the knee and elbow joints. These joints can move backward and forward in one plane like a hinge, but they cannot move in a circle like the ball and socket joints. You cannot swing your forearm about on a pivot at the elbow as you can your whole arm, nor will the knee joint bend in every direction as does the joint at the hip.

Serrated joints

Serrated joints do not move. The bones having serrated joints are fitted tightly together so that they form practically one bone. We find this kind of joint illustrated in the way the bones of the skull are put together.

Ligaments

The joints of the body are not held together by rivets, pins or bolts as are the joints of a machine, but by bands of very tough tissue placed about a joint in such a way as to allow it to move freely, although the bones are all the time held firmly together. These bands are called *ligaments*. Ligaments are much better than bolts or pegs would be, because they stretch a little, and thus prevent the breaking of the bones when the joint is put under a severe strain.

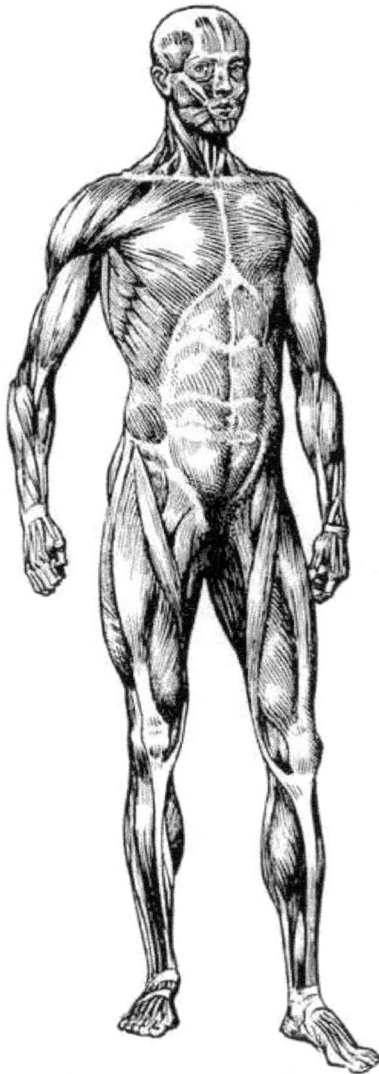

FIG. 79. The muscles.

MUSCLES AND TENDONS

What muscle is

The lean meat of any animal is composed entirely of muscle tissue. It is the function of the muscles to move the body.

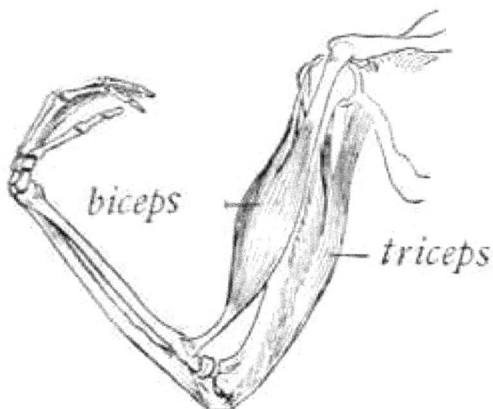

FIG. 80. The biceps muscle contracted.

How the muscles work

The muscles are nearly all attached to the bones. They are just long enough to let the joint straighten out when the muscles are at rest, but when the joint bends the muscle contracts. When a muscle contracts it becomes shorter and thicker. Sometimes it becomes very much thicker in one place. Every boy knows how much thicker the arm muscle (*biceps*) becomes when he bends his elbow hard. He calls this "showing his muscle."

Tendons

There is not room enough on most of the bones for all the muscles to be attached directly to them. Instead of being thus attached directly to the bone, they end in what we call *tendons*. These tendons are hard and strong, and a very small tendon will lift as much without breaking as quite a large muscle. The muscles are soft and would have to be attached over a large area in order to secure the required strength. The tendons, being so much stronger than the muscles, can be attached to a very small area and yet secure the same amount of power as would result from attaching the muscle itself.

The tendons pass directly into the periosteum, the thick, strong covering of the bones. So strong is this attachment that the bone will often break before the tendon will pull loose.

: The skin as an armor

The entire body is covered with skin, which regulates the heat of the body and acts as an armor against blows and cuts which would otherwise injure the delicate nerves and blood vessels beneath. It also serves to some extent to keep out the germs of disease. The skin appears to be smooth, but if you examine it through a strong magnifying glass you will see that it is divided into little areas. The dividing lines do not run straight, however, and the areas are not square like those you find on a checkerboard.

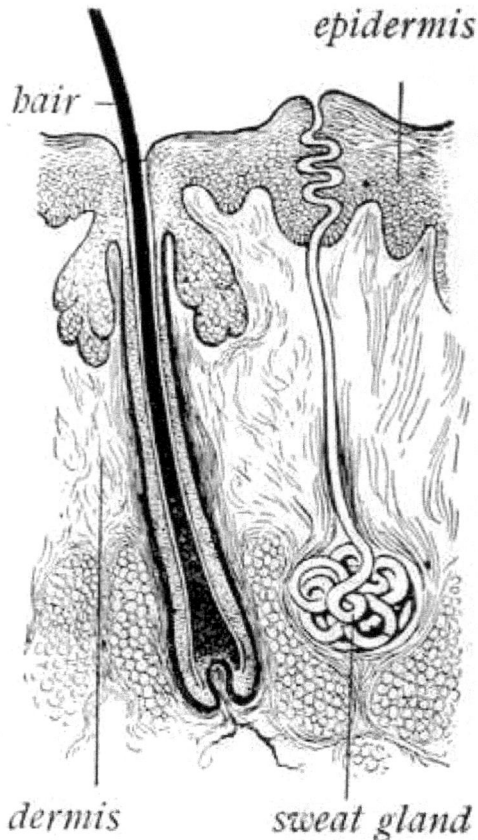

FIG. 81. A section of the skin, highly magnified.

: Sweat glands

After looking at the skin with a strong magnifying glass you will think that you must have seen all its irregularities, but if you will look at it with a powerful microscope you will find out many other things. In the first place you will see many little openings in the skin. These little openings make the ridges which divide the skin into little areas. Some of the openings are *sweat glands*, and there is always some perspiration coming out of them. When you are very warm you can see, without the aid of the glass, the drops of perspiration as they come out on the surface of the skin. When you are not very warm you cannot see these drops of perspiration, but they are nevertheless coming out all the time. When the perspiration comes so slowly that you cannot see it, it is called *insensible perspiration*.

Hair

The whole body is covered with hair. You can see the hair on your head and some of the hair on your arms and the backs of your hands, but most of the hair on the body is so fine that you cannot see it without a microscope. Each of the fine hairs on the body has a root that goes through the skin just as the root from each hair on your head goes through it.

Sebaceous glands

Opening into the little pockets in which the hairs stand, are glands that secrete a kind of oily material. They are called *sebaceous glands* or *follicles*. Sometimes these follicles become stopped up; then the material they secrete becomes thick and cheesy, and the little black points appear on the skin which we call *blackheads*. The white matter which comes out of these blackheads is merely the secretion of the glands from which the water has been absorbed, leaving the solid or cheesy portion.

Nails

There is a part of the skin that we do not usually think of as skin. We mean the *nails*. The finger nails and the toe nails do not look like the rest of the skin of the body, but they are made of just the same kind of cells. The cells of the nails are flat, dead, and closely packed together. There are no sweat glands, or sebaceous glands, or any hairs in the nails.

THE DIGESTIVE SYSTEM

The alimentary canal

The digestive system is the part of our bodies in which the food we eat is so changed that it can be made use of by the little cells in the body. It is composed of a long canal with many parts and enlargements, each part necessary for a certain required work. This canal as a whole is called the *alimentary canal*.

Teeth

The mouth does the first part of the work for the digestive system. Here we find the teeth, which are used for grinding the food. The teeth are composed of three parts, the *head* (or *crown*), the *neck* and the *root*. The head, or crown, is very hard. Each tooth is hollow, and in the hollow portion there are nerves and blood vessels.

The salivary glands

Opening into the mouth are three pairs of glands known as *salivary glands*. One pair of glands is located just above the angle of the jaw. It is these glands that become swollen when we have mumps. Another pair of glands is placed just inside the jaw bone, near the root of the tongue, and the third pair is located under the tongue. These three pairs of glands secrete the saliva which moistens the food and aids in digesting the starch.

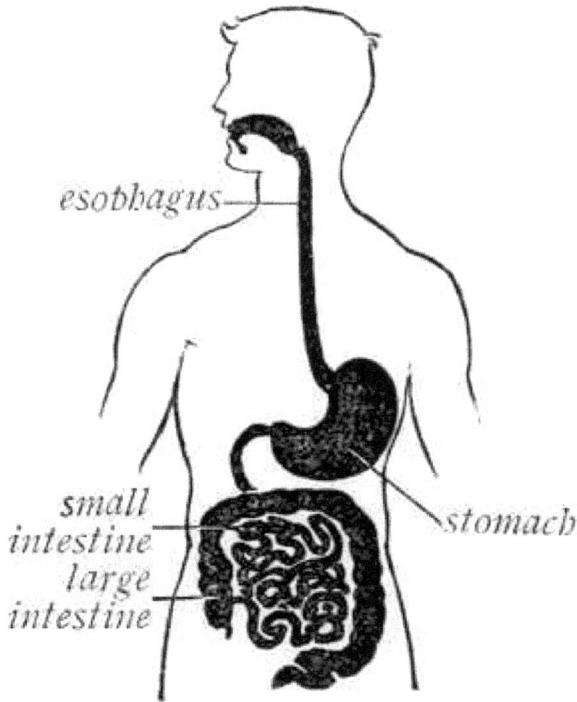

FIG. 82. The alimentary canal.

The food passes from the mouth; through a passage called the *esophagus*, or gullet, to the *stomach*.

The stomach

The stomach is one of the enlarged parts of the alimentary canal. Its walls are quite thick, and in these walls are thousands of little glands. These glands secrete a fluid called *gastric juice*. When the food enters the stomach it is held there for a long time, and the walls of the stomach squeeze upon it so that the food is mixed with the gastric juice until every bit of it that will be of any use to the body has become fluid in character. Not only does the gastric juice make the food liquid, but it acts on it and changes some of it so that it will be suitable for use by the little cells of the body. As fast as the food is made liquid by the juices of the stomach it is allowed to pass into the intestine through an opening called the *pyloric opening*.

The intestine is a long, narrow, twisting and turning tube that is divided into two principal parts, the large and small intestine. In the walls of the intestine are many little glands that secrete a fluid that helps in digesting the food. Two fluids, one made by the liver, the other by the pancreas, are brought into the intestine by two small tubes, which come together in the wall of the intestine six or seven inches below the pyloric opening. These fluids perform a very important part in the digestion of all the different foodstuffs.

Villi and lymphatics

Besides the little glands in the walls of the intestine there are many thousands of little finger-like projections standing up from the walls. These are called *villi*. Each villus has in it very small vessels, into which the food passes after it has been digested. These vessels are of two sorts: blood vessels, which take up the digested starch and proteid foods, and another sort known as *lymphatics*, which take up the fats. All the lymphatics combine into a single vessel which empties into the great vein at the base of the neck. Thus the fatty foods pass into the blood and are mingled with the food materials taken up directly by the blood vessels.

CIRCULATION OF THE BLOOD

Two kinds of blood vessels

There are two kinds of blood vessels in the body. We call them *arteries* and *veins*. The arteries serve to carry the blood from the heart to all parts of the body, and the veins serve to carry the blood back to the heart. The heart is really a part of the blood vessels, half of each side being like the veins and half like the arteries.

Arteries and veins

The walls of the arteries are thicker than those of the veins. Two sets of arteries leave the heart, one from each side. The artery that starts from the right side of the heart goes to the lungs and carries *venous blood*, which has a very poor supply of oxygen and is full of impurities. We call this the *pulmonary artery*. The artery that leaves the left side of the heart goes to all parts of the body but the lungs and carries *arterial blood*, which has much more oxygen and is much more free from impurities.

Capillaries

If we follow the blood as it circulates we will see how it reaches all parts of the body. The big artery that leaves the left side of the heart divides into smaller and smaller arteries until there are branches going to every part of the body. These branches keep dividing until they are so small that we call them *arterioles*, and these little arterioles again divide and become so small that we call them *capillaries*.

Changes in the blood

While the blood is passing through the arterioles and the capillaries, something is happening to it. The little cells with which these small vessels come in contact have been taking the oxygen and the nourishing material out of the blood. At the same time they have been putting something into the blood. In place of the oxygen they have been putting in carbon dioxid and in place of the nourishing material they have been putting in the worn-out materials from the cells. As the blood passes through certain parts of the body, such as the kidneys, the worn-out materials from the cells are taken out of the blood and sent out of the body. The carbon dioxid is left in the blood until it goes to the lungs.

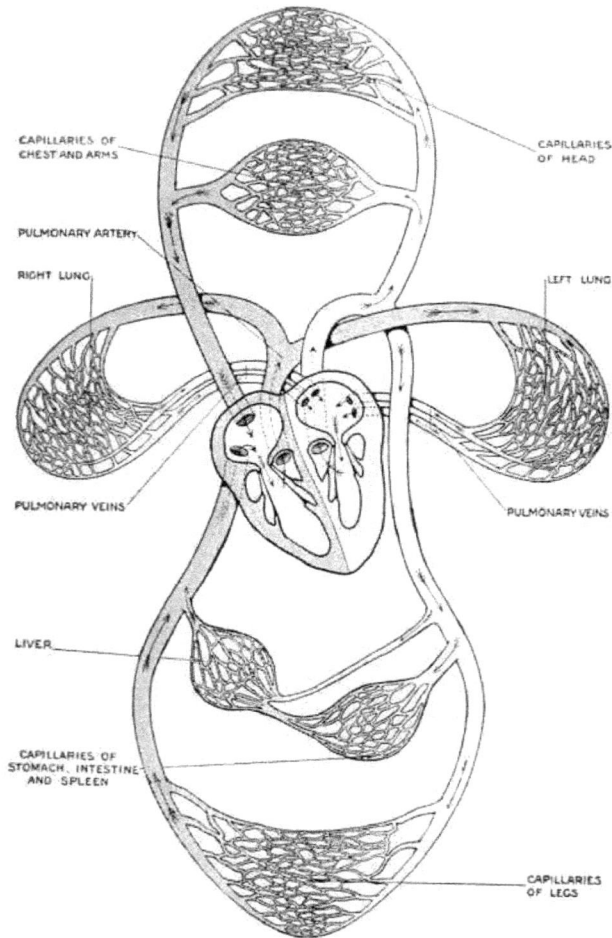

FIG. 83. The white vessels represent the circulation of the arterial blood; the gray, the circulation of the venous blood.

Venous blood

The blood has now been followed to the capillaries, where oxygen and nourishing material have been taken out of it, and where something else has been added to it. As we follow a little capillary, we find that instead of dividing again, it joins others and gradually grows larger. As these blood vessels grow larger the walls do not become so thick as the walls of the arteries of the same size. These larger vessels formed by the union of capillaries are called *veins*. In other words, the veins are simply continuations of the arteries that have divided into extremely small branches and have now come together again. The blood which has been changed is now called *venous blood*. It has much less oxygen in it, but has received a great deal of carbon dioxid. The veins continue to come together, until finally they form a single large vein which empties into the upper half of the right side of the heart. From there the blood is driven into the lower half of the right side of the heart and thence to the pulmonary artery, which goes to the lungs. The blood is not changed in the heart, so what goes into the pulmonary artery is still venous blood.

Arterial blood

The blood goes straight from the heart to the lungs and there it is changed into arterial blood. The change consists in taking oxygen from the air and giving off carbon dioxid to the air. From the lungs the blood goes through the capillaries again into the veins, the small capillaries in the lungs uniting to form the pulmonary veins. These veins finally unite into one vein that empties into the upper half of the left side of the heart, and from there the blood goes to the lower half of the same side. The blood has now reached its starting point and is ready to begin its journey again. The journey of the blood is as follows:

Entire circulation

From the right side of the heart to the arteries; from arteries into arterioles; from arterioles to capillaries; from capillaries into veins; from veins into the heart; from the heart to the lungs; and from the lungs back to the heart again.

THE RESPIRATORY SYSTEM

Use of the respiratory system

That portion of the body by which we breathe is called the respiratory system. This system is composed of the *nasal passage*, the *pharynx*, the *larynx*, the *trachea*, the *bronchi*, and the *lungs*. The mouth is not a part of the respiratory system; we should never breathe through our mouths.

The use of the nose in breathing

As the air passes through the nasal passage it is warmed and moistened, and a great deal of dust and dirt is taken out of it. Thus the nasal passage serves to warm, to moisten, and to clean the air we breathe, and is a very important part of the respiratory system, since either cold or dry air is very irritating to the lungs.

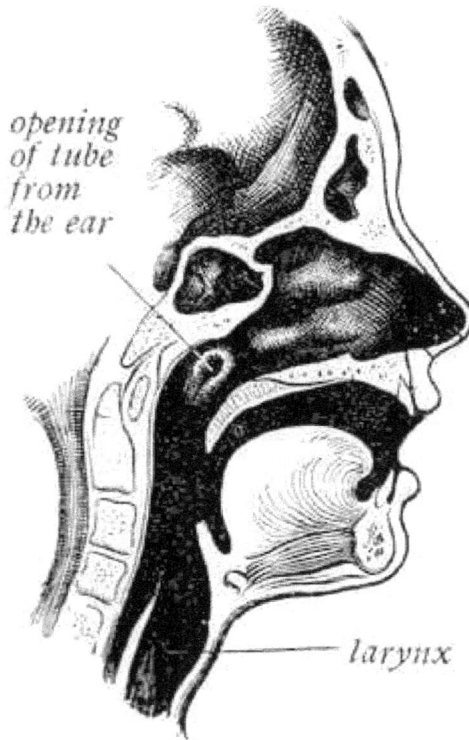

opening of tube from the ear

larynx

FIG. 84. The air passages of the head and throat.

Pharynx, larynx, and trachea

There is only one tube leading from the back of the nasal passage to the lungs. Different parts of this tube are given different names. The pharynx is that part that extends from the back of the nose to the vocal chords. The larynx is the part of the throat where the vocal chords are located. We sometimes call it the "Adam's apple." It is very prominent in some men, but seldom noticeable in women. The trachea is the part of the tube leading down from the larynx. At the lower end of the trachea the tube divides into two parts that we call the bronchi, one leading to each lung.

The bronchi

The bronchi carry the air from the trachea to the lungs. They divide again and again until they become so small that there is a branch for each little air cell in the lungs.

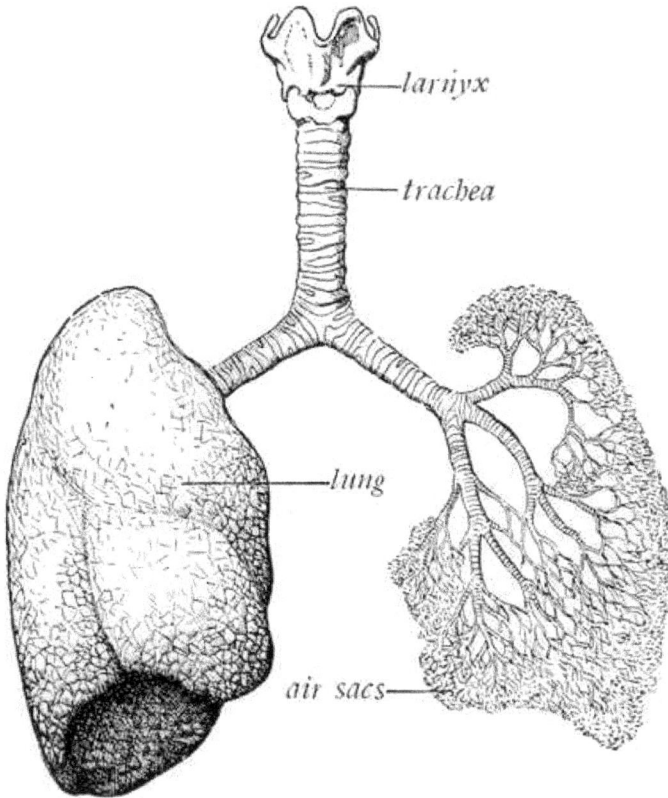

FIG. 85. The lungs.

The lungs are the most important part of the respiratory system. They are made up of lobes. There are two lobes in the left lung and three in the right. Each lobe is divided into *lobules*, which means small lobes. Each lobule is divided into air spaces. In these air spaces, or cells, the work of the lungs is performed.

Air cells

The capillaries run in the thin walls of the air spaces. The walls of these fine blood vessels are so very thin that the air in the air cells comes in almost direct contact with the blood in the vessels. While the blood is passing through the vessels in the walls of the air spaces, something happens to both the blood and the air. The air we take into our lungs contains a great deal of oxygen and very little carbon dioxid. The air that comes out of our lungs contains a great deal of carbon dioxid and much less oxygen. In other words, the oxygen from the air goes into the blood, and the carbon dioxid from the blood goes out into the air.

Necessity of pure air

If the air we breathe is not pure and does not contain enough oxygen, the blood cannot get all the oxygen we need, and the cells of the body become sick and die. If, when we breathe, we do not fill each little air cell in our lungs with air, a great deal of the blood sent to the lungs for oxygen cannot get it. If we wear very tight clothing we cannot take a full breath and hence cannot fill all the air spaces with air. If the air spaces in the lungs are not filled, the blood does not get the oxygen it needs, as there is no other place in the body to get it.

THE EYE AND THE EAR

The eye compared to a camera

The eye is one of the most important organs in the body and also one of the most delicate. It is very much like a camera.

The cornea and the sclera

When you look at an eye you are likely to think that the front of it is blue or brown. The colored part is not the front of the eye. If you look at the eye from the side you will see that there is a curved part in front of the colored part and that the curved part is perfectly clear. This curved clear part of the eye we call the *cornea*. The cornea connects with the white part of the eye, and this white part extends all around the rest of the eye, except at a small point in the back where the *optic nerve* comes through. This white part we call the *sclera*.

Aqueous humor

The space between the cornea and the colored part of the eye is filled with a clear fluid that is called the *aqueous humor*, which means watery fluid. The space occupied by this fluid is called the *anterior chamber* of the eye.

The iris, which is the colored portion of the eye, is a curtain that is hung between the anterior and posterior chambers of the eye. It prevents any light getting into the posterior chamber except that which passes through a round hole in the iris called the *pupil*. The pupil grows larger or smaller according to the amount of light needed by the eye. If you look away from a bright light at something in the dark, the pupil grows larger; if you look back at the light, it grows smaller. You can see this in a hand mirror.

Lens

Behind the pupil is a clear mass shaped like a very strong magnifying glass. This is the *lens*. The lens causes to be formed on the back of the eye a clear picture of whatever you are looking at. When you focus a camera, you move the back towards or away from the lens. When you focus your eye you cannot move the back of the eye, but you can make the lens more or less convex as may be needed to make a clear picture.

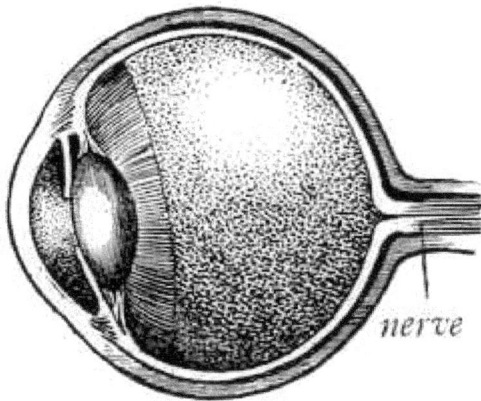

nerve

FIG. 86. A cross-section of the eye.

Vitreous humor

Behind the iris and the lens, we find the posterior chamber of the eye. This occupies by far the greater portion of the ball and corresponds to the dark chamber of a camera. This chamber is filled with a clear fluid called the *vitreous humor*, which means jelly-like fluid. It is a clear, gelatinous substance.

The retina and the optic nerve

The optic nerve enters the eyeball from the back and spreads its fibers out in a thin membrane called the *retina*, which corresponds to the sensitive plate in a camera. The lens focuses on the retina the image of any object you look at. The impression made on the minute nerve endings in the retina is carried by the optic nerve fibers to the brain. When this impression reaches the brain we see the object.

Movements of the eye

Each eye has six muscles that turn it in whatever direction you want to look. These muscles are very delicate, and for true sight they must be exactly adjusted. If the muscles on one side of the eye are stronger than those on the other side, you will be cross-eyed or wall-eyed. If one of the muscles in one eye is stronger than the corresponding muscle in the other eye, it pulls the eyeball out of place and you "see double."

The use of the outer ear

The portion of the ear that you see on the side of your head has as much to do with hearing as the outer rim of the horn into which you speak has to do with making a record for the phonograph. You know that the record is really made at the little end of the horn, while the big end simply collects the sound. The outside portion of the ear simply collects sounds, and the real hearing is done with the portion of the ear that is not seen.

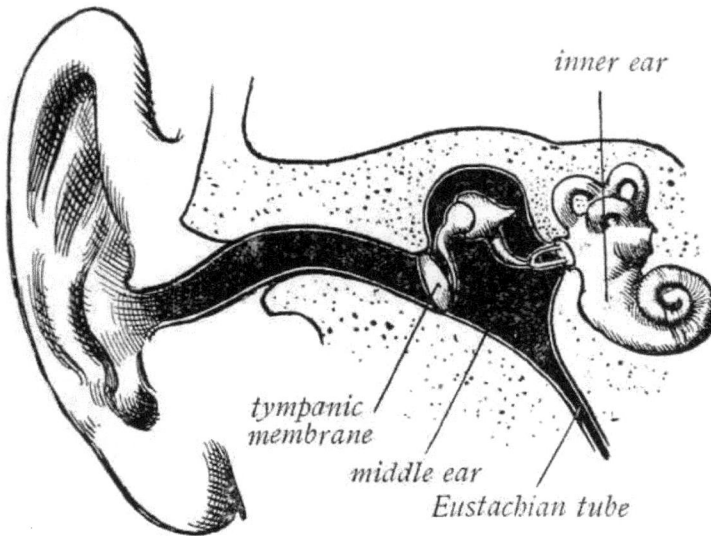

FIG. 87. The ear, showing the outer, middle, and the inner part.

The outer ear connects with the short tube that leads to the *drum*, which is a thin membrane that separates the middle ear from the outer ear. This drum does not have so much to do with hearing as is supposed. To have a hole in the drum does not mean that you cannot hear.

The middle ear

The middle ear is that portion which is just inside the drum. In this we find a chain of little bones. The one attached to the drum is shaped much like a hammer, and is called the *malleus*, which means mallet or hammer. The next one is shaped like an anvil and is called *incus*, which means anvil, and the third is called *stapes*, which means stirrup. The flat part of the stapes fits into a small opening that leads to the internal ear.

The inner ear

The internal ear is shaped like a snail shell. It makes several turns, which are hollow like the ends of a conch shell. In these channels the nerve that receives the impressions made by the sounds is distributed. This nerve carries the impressions to the brain.

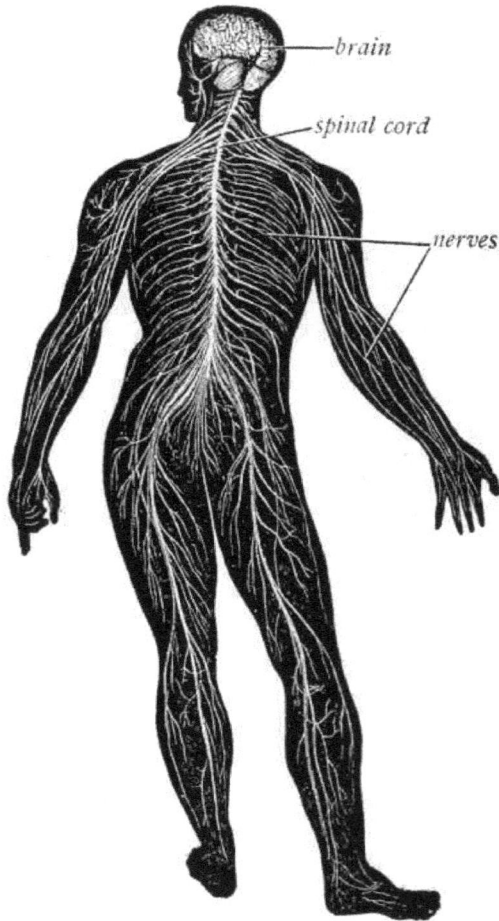

FIG. 88. The nervous system.

THE NERVOUS SYSTEM

Importance of the nervous system

This system is so important in its use and so difficult to understand in its details, that a description of it should have more space than can be given in this summary. Can you imagine having no feeling and being unable to move? This would be your condition if you had no nerves.

Nerves compared to telegraph system

Briefly, the nerves might be called the telegraph system of the body. There is a great central station called the brain where messages are received and sent out; there are many sub-stations that make up the spinal cord. Twelve great nerves pass directly from the brain to the body; all others pass from the spinal cord.

Extent of nervous system

Every nerve leaving these centres divides and sub-divides into little threads as the arteries divide and sub-divide into arterioles and capillaries, until every part of the body—every muscle and part of the skin—has its nerve.

Voluntary and reflex action

Every time you *choose* to move your hand, your brain sends to the necessary muscles an instantaneous order to act. This is called *voluntary action*. If you put your finger against a hot stove you jerk it away before you could have time to *choose* to do it. This happens as an order from a sub-station and is called *reflex action*.

Messages travel both ways and it is necessary that the nervous connection with every part of the body remain unbroken, and important that the nervous condition be kept healthy.

NOTES TO THE TEACHER

A false delicacy has often prevented the teaching of vital lessons to growing children. The day is how at hand when foolish sentiment must no longer prevent the spread of any knowledge which is necessary to exterminate the plagues that have afflicted the race.

In chapters 17, 18, 19 and 32, unpleasant facts are given in plain language. They are facts that parents do not teach their children and that most teachers will not frankly treat with classes in a school. Though they are disagreeable to discuss, they are essential for children of school age to know. Now that the dependence of public health upon personal hygiene is recognized, personal habits and sanitary conditions are more frankly dealt with than formerly.

It is an excellent thing occasionally, to have one or two points of an assigned lesson answered in writing. Any topic that the teacher may think advisable to treat in this manner may be discussed on paper at the beginning of the recitation, five or six minutes being allowed for that purpose. Even a whole chapter may be assigned to be studied with a view of answering in writing the questions at the end of the chapter. The written test can then take the place of the usual oral recitation. This method is suggested to the teacher who hesitates to discuss orally certain plain but essential facts.

Chapter 32 on the Spread and Prevention of Consumption can be treated with best results orally, if the pupils are first made to *feel* the great danger of consumption and to realize the possibility of preventing the vast havoc wrought by that dread disease. The attitude of teacher and pupils should be that while the discussion may be disagreeable, the disgusting habits referred to in the text are so commonly practised that unless their dangers are taught this disease can never be wiped out.

FOOTNOTES:

Bujar and Baier state that the nourishing power of bacon is represented by 2,767, while the nourishing power of butter is represented by 2,610.

The cleaning out of these cemented vaults is an exceedingly unpleasant task. Some prefer to have a strong, water-tight box placed under the closet seats. When this box is nearly full, it can be removed to some place where fertilizer is needed, and there emptied, the contents being plowed into the ground. In order to make this task as simple as possible, it is a good plan to put the box on skids, and have a heavy strip in one end with a bolt and ring through it, so that a horse can be hitched to the box to draw it away. If a little dry earth or lime is put into the box each day, there will be no unpleasant odor.

The teacher should demonstrate the action of acids and alkalies on a solution of litmus.

At the request of many practical teachers the author has appended this brief summary of anatomy. The material is intended to be used for reference or to be assigned as lessons in connection with the chapters of the book, at the discretion of the teacher.

Milton Keynes UK
Ingram Content Group UK Ltd.
UKHW030624061024
449204UK00004B/350

9 789362 510273